The New Culture of Dementia Care

Edited by
Tom Kitwood
and Sue Benson

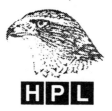

HPL

Hawker Publications
Journal of Dementia Care
in association with
Bradford Dementia Group

First published in 1995 by
Hawker Publications Ltd
13 Park House
140 Battersea Park Road
London SW11 4NB

British Library Cataloguing in Publication Data

A catalogue record for this book is available
from the British Library

ISBN 1 874790 17 5

Key Words: *Dementia, Care, Alzheimer's disease, Culture, Training*

Design by
Richard Souper

Typeset by
Hawker Publications

Printed and bound in Great Britain by
The Book Factory, London

Contents

Contributors   4

Introduction: Widening our vision of dementia care   5
Alison Froggatt

1. Cultures of care: tradition and change   7
Tom Kitwood

2. A challenge to stage theories of dementia   12
Janet Bell and Iain McGregor

3. Sharing the care: towards new forms of communication   15
Jean Tobin

4. The beginnings of a new culture in care   19
Bob Woods

5. People with dementia can communicate – if we are able to hear   24
Brigitte A Frank

6. Well-being, personality and residential care   30
Sean Buckland

7. Sexuality and sexual needs of the person with dementia   35
Carole Archibald

8. Broadening our approach to spirituality   40
Elizabeth Barnett

9. The genetics of Alzheimer's disease: rethinking the questions   44
Andrea Capstick

10. Support through human contact for family carers   49
Errolyn Bruce

11. Backs to the wall? Day care within the new culture   54
Paul Cunningham and Jane Kesterton

12. People with dementia in sheltered housing   58
Tracy Petre

13. Involving volunteers in care provision   62
Rosas Mitchell

14. A new pattern of life: re-assessing the role of occupation and activities   66
Tessa Perrin

15. Mapping the advance of the new culture in dementia care   70
Linda Fox

16. Strategies for training and organisational change   75
Brenda Bowe and Buz Loveday

Index   80

Contributors

Carole Archibald RGN, HV, BA is senior fieldworker at the Dementia Services Development Centre, University of Stirling. She worked as a specialist health visitor, with people with dementia and their carers, at the Royal Edinburgh Hospital before taking up post at the University of Stirling in 1989.

Elizabeth Barnett BA, DipSS is Dementia Care Mapping project manager, Bath Mental Health Care NHS Trust. She is presently writing up her PhD in Social Policy (dementia care) at Bath University and is an Associate of the Bradford Dementia Group. She is a Quaker, and recently spent three months at Woodbrooke College in Birmingham following the Quaker studies course.

Janet Bell and **Iain McGregor** opened Spring Mount residential home, Bradford, in 1987. Before this Janet Bell RMN, RGN, CPN had worked in the NHS for eighteen years, nine of them as a community psychiatric nurse specialising in dementia care. Iain McGregor CQSW, Certificate in Group Psychotherapy worked for twelve years for social services, in hospitals and in the community, as a specialist caseworker in dementia care.

Sue Benson BA, RGN is editor of the *Journal of Dementia Care*.

Brenda Bowe and **Buz Loveday** work in Hackney, East London, in a Mental Illness Specific Grant funded project – the Outreach Resource Team – which provides training, support, counselling, consultancy, groupwork development, Dementia Care Mapping and other services for anyone in the borough who works with/cares for people with dementia. Brenda Bowe DipCOT is a qualified occupational therapist who has worked as a fieldworker and manager in several London boroughs. Buz (Rosalind) Loveday is trained as a counsellor.

Errolyn Bruce BA, MA has a first degree in psychology and an MA in social and community work. She has worked in community work, research and further education, and has had a lifelong interest in health and illness. She is now community support worker with Bradford Dementia Group.

Sean Buckland BSc is a research psychologist with Bradford Dementia Group. Previously employed in Portsmouth as an assistant psychologist doing hospital based research and interventions with persons with severe dementia, as well as quality assurance and community work, his current research aims to identify factors associated with the well-being and ill-being of persons with dementia living in residential settings.

Andrea Capstick BA (Interdisciplinary Human Studies) is project officer (research) with Bradford Dementia Group, researching the social and ethical aspects of the genetics of Alzheimer's disease.

Paul Cunningham is manager of a centre offering seven-day provision for individuals with dementia, for Leeds City Council Department of Social Services. He has worked in residential and day care for eight years, and is an advanced dementia care mapper and evaluator.

Linda Fox BA (Interdisciplinary Human Studies) is administrator for Bradford Dementia Group. She also carries out evaluations using the dementia care mapping method on behalf of the group, and co-facilitates the weekly *Focus on dementia* carers' support programme. Her previous experience includes work in formal care settings.

Brigitte A Frank BA, MA is nursing assistant and residents' affairs officer for Riverside Mental Health Trust and an associate of the Bradford Dementia Group. Her chapter is based on research undertaken as a PhD student and research assistant (Discourse Analysis) at the University of Surrey/Roehampton Institute.

Alison Froggatt BA, MA, AIMSW, formerly lecturer in social work at Bradford University, is now a consultant and trainer in work with elderly people, especially for church groups. She is an associate of Bradford Dementia Group and member of the Dementia Working Group, Christian Council on Ageing.

Jane Kesterton BA is manager of a multi-cultural centre for Leeds City Council Department of Social Services. She has worked in residential and day care for eight years, and is currently an advanced dementia care mapper and evaluator, and associate of the Bradford Dementia Group.

Tom Kitwood BA, MSc, PhD, AFBPS, CPsychol. is senior lecturer in psychology at the University of Bradford, and leader of Bradford Dementia Group.

Rosas Mitchell BSocSc, Dipl. Applied Social Studies is project worker (dementia initiative), for social work services at Bellsdyke Hospital, Larbert, Scotland. She trained in social work in Birmingham and Glasgow, specialising in the areas of mental health and learning difficulty. More recently she has worked as a co-ordinator in a Crossroads Care Attendant Scheme, before taking up her present post.

Tessa Perrin MSc, DipCOT is employed by Essex County Council Social Services Department as senior practitioner occupational therapist, and has specialised in dementia care in the residential and day care sector. She is currently on secondment to the Bradford Dementia Research Group, where she is investigating the role of occupations in the treatment of those with advanced dementia.

Tracy Petre BSc is a research student with Bradford Dementia Group, researching the effects of dementia on sheltered housing today, and the ways in which negative effects can be removed and positive ones enhanced. She completed a degree in psychology at the University of Central Lancashire.

Jean Tobin MPhil is an associate of Bradford Dementia Group. She was formerly principal lecturer in education studies, Bradford and Ilkley Community College, and retired early to care for her mother with dementia at home for five years. Jean has been a member of various carer support groups, and has been involved in the training of dementia care staff, and in teaching and using dementia care mapping.

Bob Woods MA, MSc, FBPsS, CPsychol. is senior lecturer in psychology, University College London. He began working with older people with dementia over 20 years ago, first as a nursing assistant in a psychogeriatric ward, and then as a clinical psychologist. In addition to his academic post, he is also currently head of psychology services for older people with the Camden & Islington Community Health Services NHS Trust.

Introduction: Widening our vision of dementia care

ALISON FROGGATT

*I*n the last few years there has been a surge of interest in dementia. Partly because of and partly in spite of the changing welfare scene, community care and the closing of the asylums, dementia care has come out of the closet. The back wards in geriatric hospitals are no longer in use, and many new forms of care provision are being tried out. Amid all these changes, there is serious interest in how to care well for people with chronic illnesses, including those with brain failure.

In 1994 awareness and interest in new ways of working reached a point where the Bradford Dementia Group, led by Tom Kitwood, held a conference that proved to be a milestone in the endeavour to draw together current knowledge and experience of treating dementia in a person-centred way. In order to disseminate the insights that were shared there, it was decided to publish a book based on the conference addresses and workshops. The book forms a staging post in the journey of discovery into understanding what people go through in the processes involved in the conditions described as the dementias. Two chapters, by people who have joined Bradford Dementia Group since the conference, have been added. This in itself is an example of the rapid development of understanding in this field.

The new culture of dementia care has been in the making for several years. About ten years ago a number of us, drawn from different professional backgrounds – psychology, medicine, social work and community psychiatric nursing – began to ask each other "What is it like to have dementia?" "What are people with dementia going through?" Before then, by far the greater part of concern had been with the needs of carers. Our discussions in Bradford reflected the beginning of a new awareness growing throughout Britain, and indeed the world at large.

The growth of understanding

There were glimmers of understanding, and a process of collecting clues began. At that stage there was a gradually increasing awareness of what was being experienced. Now our shared understanding, underpinned by research, observation and further reflection, has shown that a new culture of dementia care is possible and desirable, even essential. We have found that we can begin to describe it from different perspectives – represented in the chapters of this book.

Tom Kitwood provides a theoretical framework which has enabled people to find a voice. His paper shows the development of his ideas into this new culture of dementia care, which has been rethought and reworked from much richer and wider database than that used in the technical account of dementia.

I have been involved with Spring Mount residential home since its inception. Here Janet Bell and Iain McGregor offer both a challenge to the generally accepted ways of viewing dementia, and an environment which shows the uniqueness of persons. Their home is a living example of what can be achieved through a different culture of care. The good practice which they have developed over the past years in Spring Mount now allows them to share their ideas with considerable confidence. They have shown that people with dementia can really flourish if they are given an environment that offers a sense of well-being and makes the most of their potential to develop.

As a balance to the work of paid carers, Jean Tobin has much to contribute to our understanding of how family carers feel, the part they want to play in sharing care, and the significant burden they bear in personal and economic terms. She demonstrates the importance of paid carers and family carers cooperating together in a mutual endeavour.

Bob Woods shows how there has been concern about the personhood of those with dementia for a number of years and in different contexts. Many people were aware that the person with dementia was struggling to maintain self respect, but even skilled practitioners lacked the voice, the language, and the confidence to share their ideas with each other. In his chapter Woods gives us the framework from which to assess this new culture, showing us the roots of it, located in the best forms of earlier care such as active stimulation, reality orientation, reminiscence and validation therapy.

In discussing issues of communication, Brigitte Frank reminds us that despite all that has been written on what people with dementia cannot do or say, their communication abilities are greater than we may realise. Elizabeth Barnett, writing of spiritual aspects in dementia care challenges the superficiality and materialism of the present time. She affirms that people with dementia are fully human, spiritual beings with spiritual needs.

In exploring the genetic aspects of dementia, Andrea Capstick points out how easy it is for for scientific and technical research to press forward without concern for social and ethical issues. It is vitally important, she argues, to bring genetic research into a human frame.

Drawing on her work in developing support groups for carers of people with dementia, Errolyn Bruce emphasises how much systematic and sensitive support is needed and valued. To offer this is a much bigger undertaking than is generally realised. Tracy Petre discusses the issue of dementia in sheltered housing. She concludes that the well-being of people with dementia depends primarily on the overall quality of life in the sheltered scheme.

Sean Buckland explores the issues of quality of care and well-being in residential settings; particularly how we take the variety of personalities into account. Jane Kesterton and Paul Cunningham tell us about their experience in day care, and the measures they have taken to help bring about a new culture. Carol Archibald's chapter discusses the complex issue of sexuality, recognising that people with dementia are sexual beings like all of us, and giving practical guidance on developing a positive approach.

Rosas Mitchell draws on her work with volunteers to show how creative and innovative practice can involve volunteers in a variety of ways. There is much good work here on which the new culture of care can draw. Occupational therapist Tessa Perrin invites us to think more deeply about the nature and meaning of occupation; purposive activity, she argues, is central to our human life.

A chapter exploring the advance of the new culture of dementia care, using evidence from dementia care mapping (DCM) has been contributed by Linda Fox. DCM has been a valuable instrument in the spread of the new culture, as well as a quality assurance measure. Finally Buz Loveday and Brenda Bowe, arguing the importance of training at all levels in an organisation, show that the problems of bringing about radical change go very deep.

Despite the wide variety of professional perspectives and contexts demonstrated in these chapters, they cannot claim to cover all aspects of dementia care – far from it. There are many other avenues to explore in future: the needs of members in extended families; the care offered to black and ethnic minority communities. The particular needs of younger sufferers, or where there is a strong genetic form of dementia, require special understanding.

Nurturing growth of the new culture

To try to bring about widespread and lasting change in attitudes and practice in dementia care is no easy matter. To make progress requires a huge and sustained input of energy from many people. A significant obstacle, and a reason for the traditionally low priority of dementia care, is the fear and avoidance the subject provokes in so many of us.

Training in the ideas and practice of the new culture must be concerned not only with professionals but a range of people in the community, including neighbours, volunteers, and those offering day care or family sitting services. These workers, and all family carers, will need help in entering this new kind of care with the extra demands it brings – not least of which is the challenge to personal growth in the carer.

We can share this new culture with those grappling with other disabling conditions. People with learning difficulties, Parkinson's disease, multiple sclerosis, for example – all could benefit from a climate of care that includes understanding of their personality and autobiography as well as their family and the setting in which they now live.

With uncertainty over the future of NHS long-term care, we are seeing a boom in new specialist provision for people with severe dementia. It is essential that the ideas of the new culture are fed in to these projects at the planning stage, to counteract any temptation to go for technical solutions, ignoring what human skill, insight and warmth can offer. We would argue that a larger proportion of financial resources should be spent on the initial training of staff and further staff development and support, for example. The new culture does make particular emotional, intellectual and spiritual demands on staff, as well as the physical ones more usually expected. It is essential that organisations in this field of care provide ways to take good care of all the needs of their staff.

Supremely valuable work

The ideas and suggestions put forward in these pages reflect changes that have already been brought about in practice. The picture of dementia is thrown wide open. No longer can it be seen merely as a nasty disease process which has unfortunately struck a family member. More and more, it is now being viewed as a complex interaction of neurological and psychological changes, affected markedly by the social and emotional environment in which each person lives.

Dementia care in the new culture requires understanding afresh for each affected person. This makes considerable demands on all concerned, to nourish and sustain the individual as someone known and loved, who has lived a fruitful and competent life in earlier years. We hope you will find stimulation and sustenance in these chapters, and recognition of the supremely valuable and skilled work which dementia care entails.

Alison Froggatt
Bradford, April 1995

CHAPTER ONE | Cultures of care: tradition and change

TOM KITWOOD

The historical background to the old culture of care is traced in outline. Ten key points of contrast between the old and the new cultures of dementia care are given and explained.

*O*ne of the most striking facts about dementia care at the present time is the tremendous variety of its quality. When we spend some time in a really good care environment, several things are likely to impress us. Those who have dementia are very much alive, responsive, relating to each other, making their presence felt; there is the sense that a lot is going on. The staff seem to be enjoying what they are doing; they are satisfied, relaxed and free. Not all is happiness and peace, of course – but there is vitality, energy, inspiration.

However, we also know environments that are very different from this. There is a sense of deadness, apathy, boredom, gloom and fear; most of those being cared for appear to have given up hope, their last resort being an occasional moan, or shout, or angry outburst. The staff are patronising, cynical, uninvolved, and even relating to each other largely in superficial ways. One way of describing this remarkable difference is to say that it represents two contrasting cultures of care.

The asylum tradition

The uncertainty that so clearly marks the present time has come about, in part, because of the breaking up of ways of dealing with the mentally infirm that were established over 300 years ago.

It was during the 17th century that the foundations of the modern European societies were firmly laid. This was the period when many nation states emerged, with more or less the boundaries we know today, and when a general way of life structured around production, trade and profit began to take form. In the cause of "efficiency" and "rationality" large numbers of obvious misfits – the mad, the deformed, beggars, witches and the flagrantly immoral – were taken out of society and put into a new kind of institution. Later these were called asylums (meaning, paradoxically, a place of safety, to describe a place where all forms of safety were imperilled).

The history of this "great confinement", as the French historian Michel Foucault has called it, unfolds in three main phases (Foucault 1967). The first was one of *bestialisation*, where the inmates were treated very much as animals in an old-fashioned zoo: crowded in wretched cages, left untended, and on view to a sensation-seeking public on high days and holidays.

There followed a phase of *moralisation*, through the main part of the 19th century, with high-minded attempts to re-create the asylum as a place of kindly re-education. Then, around the turn of our own century, came a new phase of *medicalisation*, through which many types of non-conformity were re-classified as disease. The patterns of "uncare" that we know so well in the case of dementia, are largely inherited from these different phases.

Now the asylums have closed or are closing, for reasons that are as much financial as humanistic (Murphy 1991). This does not in itself mean that those with dementia have better life prospects. For the worst possibility is that we might simply see the bad patterns of the past reconstituted: either in new and smaller institutions, many of which are in private hands, or in people's own homes as they await their so-called packages of care. Nothing, then, follows automatically from the sweeping changes that are now taking place. All that can be said is that this is a time of opportunity to do something better. Any success will be achieved through a movement contrary to the shallow, technical and money-obsessed mentality of our times.

The idea of a culture

We could define a culture as "a settled, patterned way of giving meaning to human existence in the world, and of giving structure to action within it" (Williams 1976). Three components of a culture are important for us here. First there are institutions, through which social power is clearly allocated. Second there are norms, meaning standards for behaviour, including that within the main institutions. Third, there are beliefs, both about the nature of what is, and about what ought to be. The power of a culture stems from the fact that when people are immersed in it, the framework that it provides seems self-evident. What nature is to creatures whose lives are governed by instinct, culture is to human beings, who live their lives in a world of meanings.

One point about cultures deserves special attention here. It is often thought that the actions of human beings follow their beliefs, as if by logical deduction. History, however, often gives us another picture: that the institutions arise first, with their ways of establishing power and control; then follow the beliefs, in order to create "facts" that fit in (Henriques & Hollway 1984). The Europeans colonised black peoples in their search for trade and valuable materials; later they defined these peoples as inferior, in justification of the status quo (Fanon 1967). We find such specious rationalisations in every part of human life.

So our understanding of culture needs to be enriched by an idea from psychoanalysis (Becker 1973). This is that each culture has its special way of occluding, or hiding away, parts of the truth about human existence that are too difficult or inconvenient to bear. Some cultures, perhaps, are relatively open, without strong vested interests in obscuring the truth. Others, especially those which have great disparities of power and elaborate forms of control, are deeply repressive. The "rational", masculine cultures of the Europeans, in which our patterns of so-called care are embedded, are of the latter kind.

A contrast of cultures

I wish now to draw out ten differences between the old and new cultures of dementia care. The emphasis here is on beliefs and attitudes. Behind these lie the organisations, with their power structures and their patterns of status and control.

1. Attitude to dementia care

Old culture: *Dementia care is a backwater, and deservedly so. The demands are high, but the real challenges are few. It is an area of work well suited to those who have low ability, little inspiration and few qualifications.*

Here the shadow of the asylum is clearly visible. People with dementia sometimes resemble wild beasts which cannot be controlled – they simply need "keepers"; they are incapable of receiving moral education; they are afflicted with an incurable disease. There is little that can be done for them, except to wait until they die.

New culture: *Dementia care is one of the richest areas of human work. It requires very high levels of ability, creativity and insight. In our involvement with those who have dementia we are pushing our humanity to its outer limits.*

The change to this view has been taking place for

some years now. An increasing number of people are involved in work with those who have dementia because they want to be there, because of a sense of commitment. New forms of training are needed, and a freeing of the personality from defensiveness and restraint.

2. General view of dementia

Old culture: *The primary degenerative dementias are devastating diseases of the central nervous system, in which personality and identity are progressively destroyed.*

In such a definition there is no recognition of the human environment that surrounds a person with dementia. It is as if he or she is left alone and powerless, while the degenerative process takes its course. This deeply pessimistic view is not supported by scientific evidence; it is, rather, a reflection of the kind of institutional setting in which dementia care has traditionally taken place.

New culture: *Dementing illnesses should be seen, primarily, as forms of disability. How a person is affected depends crucially on the quality of care.*

Here there is no denying of the damage that occurs to nervous tissue, or of the consequences for a person's abilities. However, matters are taken out of the negative, deterministic framework that the old culture had created, by placing the emphasis on human action. The focus is on enabling and empowering, through the provision of what is necessary to compensate for disability, and on recognising the unique way in which each person deals with his or her damaged world.

3. Ultimate source of knowledge

Old culture: *In relation to dementia, the people who possess the most reliable, valid and relevant knowledge are the doctors and the brain scientists. We should defer to them.*

Here again we see an almost superstitious belief. It is not based on any systematic review of the findings of medical science, nor an appraisal of its benefits for those who have dementia. It is rather, an inference from the structure of power. If medical science has so much power, if it attracts such vast funding, then it must be important and true; whatever knowledge we have gained through action must be trivial compared to theirs.

New culture: *In relation to dementia, the people who possess the most reliable, valid and relevant knowledge are skilled and insightful practitioners of care.*

The key point here is that those who actually do the caring have a great advantage as researchers, when compared to medical scientists. For one thing, they have far more data, because they know a person over a sustained period, with all the accompanying fluctuations of mood and action. For another, they have data concerning the whole person in everyday life: knowledge, so to speak, of the working of an exceedingly intricate system, taken as a system.

This is more valuable, in many respects, than knowledge about the functioning of minute parts; for with a system, the functioning of the whole is never ascertained by merely analysing the parts. Good caregivers are not necessarily good researchers; they may not have a framework for making sense of their knowledge. The point is that the best database is there for them, and there is no reason for them to be talked out of the knowledge that they have tested in experience.

4. Emphasis for research

Old culture: *There is not much that we can do positively for a person with dementia, until the medical breakthroughs come. Hence much more biomedical research is urgently needed.*

Beliefs of this kind underpin the enormous outlay of money and the great dedication of scientific talent to biomedical research related to dementia. Often we are presented, at a popular level, with the impression that great discoveries are just round the corner.

A closer inquiry, however, suggests that this is far from being the case. Research itself has often been allied to commercial interests, or driven by the pursuit of what is "technically sweet". Inferences drawn from research at a popular level are full of fallacy and half-truths.

New culture: *There is a great deal that we can do now, through the amplification of human insight and skill. This is the most urgent matter for research.*

The new culture certainly welcomes the genuine discoveries of brain science, when the surrounding garbage has been cleared away. It does, however, suggest that the priorities of the last 40 years have been inept, often governed more by vested interests than a concern with truth or the relief of suffering. The social psychology of dementia – how a person relates, communicates, compensates, makes sense, responds to change – is only in its infancy. Yet even now we have sufficient ground for believing that this is where many great new breakthroughs will come.

5. Us and Them

Old culture: *Those who have dementia are significantly different from the rest of us, because of their "organic mental disorder". Hence there is a legitimacy in staff having different styles of clothing, meals, crockery, chairs, toilets, etc.*

Again we see beliefs that reflect the form of life of the institution, rather than an inference from sound

research. The old-time asylum, with its imposition of power and its imperative of control, could only function by creating a massive difference between staff and inmates. If there was too much "fraternisation", all legitimacy for the system would collapse.

New culture: *Those who have dementia are equal members of the human race with the rest of us. We are all persons, and all, fundamentally, in the same boat. This should be reflected in our practice.*

The new culture, then, works to minimise difference. Let us be clear that this does not, in any sense, mean a grading down of competent people. It does, however, require all of us to own up to our areas of damage and deficit, not hiding behind a professional facade; and, on the other side, to perceive, honour, and nurture the qualities of each person with dementia, however seemingly damaged or unattractive they may be.

6. What caring involves

Old culture: *Care is concerned primarily with such matters as providing a safe environment, meeting basic needs (food, clothing, toileting, warmth, cleanliness, adequate sleep, etc), and giving physical care in a competent way.*

In other words, the old culture is involved primarily with what is obvious, external, easily managed. This was the emphasis placed in the training of several generations of nurses. Their expertise lies here. If they did in fact engage with persons, it was not on the official agenda.

New culture: *Care is concerned primarily with the maintenance and enhancement of personhood. Providing a safe environment, meeting basic needs and giving physical care are all essential, but only part of the care of the whole person.*

So the new culture sets a much larger, more interesting, more personally demanding agenda. The maintenance and enhancement of another's personhood is something that requires very delicate sensitivities, very highly developed skills, and hence new forms of preparation and training. The care of the whole person, moreover, requires carers to be whole persons too, cured of their mania for control.

7. Priorities for understanding

Old culture: *It is important to have a clear and accurate understanding of a person's impairments, especially those of cognition. The course of a dementing illness can be charted in terms of stages of decline.*

The old culture feeds on deficits, both neurological and psychological, and a tremendous amount of money, time and energy has been expended in discovering what people with dementia cannot do. All this might be helpful if it led to forms of action that would bring about improvement. Generally, however, this is not the case, and the main consequence is often further labelling. Much the same applies to those stage theories that chart a person's decline: assuming (without clear evidence) that this decline is due solely to the degeneration of nervous tissue. Stage theories are linked to scenarios of gloom and doom; it is hard to find any instance where they have led to better forms of care.

New culture: *It is important to have a clear and accurate understanding of a person's abilities, tastes, interests, values, forms of spirituality. There are as many manifestations of dementia as there are persons with dementia.*

The key point here is that while we all have deficits and impairments of some kind, we also have a marvellous capacity for overcoming them. So the new culture is concerned primarily with what a person can do and wants to do, and finding the conditions under which he or she can thrive even in the face of disability. From this perspective the classification of deficits, or placing a person in a stage sequence, has a very minor place. One has, rather, a sharpened sense of the uniqueness of the individual, each with his or her personality and life-history. Disability is fitted into that pattern, and not the other way round.

8. "Problem behaviours"

Old culture: *When a person shows problem behaviours, these must be managed skilfully and efficiently.*

Notice the language here; it is the language of control, spoken by those who have power about those who do not. It would be refreshing to hear people talk about managing the behaviour of the royalty, or our political leaders, or the super-rich tycoons and landlords. Managing the behaviour of another means a disregard of that person's own frame of reference, their struggle for life and meaning.

New culture: *All so-called problem behaviours should be viewed, primarily, as attempts at communication, related to need. It is necessary to seek to understand the message, and so to engage with the need that is not being met.*

The first thing, then, is to drop the concept of behaviour, and replace it by the concept of action. This is to recognise that each person (even when carrying severe cognitive impairments), looks for the meaning of the situation, formulates an intention, and then tries to make something happen in line with that intention.

When we re-frame the so-called problem-behaviours in this way, again and again we find that they have meaning; perhaps at first we were too narrow-minded to see it. There is no denying that we may be disturbed and annoyed by what a person with dementia is doing – and with good reason. But the new culture points to a way of finding solutions that meet the needs of all concerned.

9. Carers' feelings

Old culture: *In the process of care the key thing is to set aside our own concerns, feelings, vulnerabilities, etc, and get on with the job in a sensible, effective way.*

One great difficulty with this is that it seems to require carers to be less than the fully human beings they really are. The old culture actually encouraged people to hide behind a professional mask, to avoid facing the truth about themselves. For many carers, then, their anxiety, depression, impotence and rage remained hidden away in the shadow – exerting a negative influence but in unacknowledged ways. It is not surprising that the old culture produced so much abuse, both physical and psychological, and was accompanied by such a high degree of burn-out.

New culture: *In the process of care the key thing is to be in touch with our concerns, feelings, vulnerabilities, etc, and transform these into positive resources for our work.*

The new culture encourages us to use every part of our being. If I know my own feelings, I can engage my feeling self when I am caring for another; if I know my vulnerabilities, I can lovingly take care of these, and draw on my self-knowledge as a basis for empathy. There is no question here of a carer being overwhelmed by his or her own emotions, and so being rendered ineffectual. It is simply the invitation to be real, whole people, knowing who we are and what we bring.

10. Personhood of staff

Old culture: *Direct care staff are "servants of the organisation". It is not on the agenda of the organisation to take them really seriously, or to engage with their psychological needs.*

This view goes along naturally with the old institutions and their distribution of power. The care worker was to be some kind of combination of zoo-keeper, guard, moral tutor and medical orderly – reflecting the different phases of the asylum tradition. And since those with dementia had the lowest status of all inmates, little was either required of or given to those who looked after them.

New culture: *Direct care staff are persons. Respect for their personhood is as much on the agenda of the organisation as respect for the personhood of those who have dementia.*

This point is absolutely crucial, and recognition of it still lags far behind. Some organisations that are committed to the new culture are only part-way there: they acknowledge the need to recognise the personhood of the clients, but do not perceive accurately the necessary conditions for bringing this about. Staff can only give person-centred care to others, in the long term, if their own personhood is acknowledged and nurtured. Where this is not the case, they will revert to lower aspirations and less committed forms of practice – except for a few lonely heroes who place themselves in grave danger of exhaustion and burn-out.

The new culture, however, fosters a realistic long-term commitment, providing the means of personal renewal in the face of difficult and demanding work.

Great contrasts

The contrasts, then, between the old culture and the new appear to be very great. Sometimes when I make comparisons in this kind of way I wonder if I am exaggerating. It is all too easy to set up a "straw man" and then demolish it in order to score points.

However, just after I finished the basic preparation of what I have written here, and while I was having some doubts, an article appeared on my desk. It was from a popular magazine. The headline was *Alzheimer's – No Cure, No Help, No Hope*. There followed the dreadful story of a man who had developed a dementing illness around the age of 40, and of the burden and anguish of his wife and family. This account offered not a single ray of hope at the human level, but ended with an invitation to donate to a particular fund for neuroscientific research. Virtually every feature of the old culture, as I have set it out here, was displayed at some point in this article.

I do not wish in any way to make light of the suffering that surrounds dementia, both for those who have it and for their families and friends. But I have to say that what the article contained was not the truth as I know it, even in instances of early dementia that are just as severe. It was not the truth; it was a representation that used the concepts of the old culture. The new culture, also, does not provide "the truth"; but it does provide a very different representation, grounded in a richer range of evidence and experience.

Coming home

What, then, lies at the core of the difference between the two cultures? I think it is this. The old culture is one of alienation and estrangement. Through it we are distanced from our fellow human beings, deprived of our insight, cut off from our own vitality. The old culture is one of domination, technique, evasion and buck-passing. To enter the new culture is like coming home. We can now draw close to other human beings, accepting all that we genuinely share. We can recover confidence in our power to know, to discover, to give, to create, to love. And this homecoming is a cause for joy and celebration.

References
Foucault M (1967) *Madness and Civilization*. English Translation by Richard Howard. Tavistock, London.
Murphy E (1991) *After the Asylums*. Faber, London.
Williams R (1976) *Keywords: A Vocabulary of Culture and Society*. Fontana, London.
Henriques J, Hollway W, Urwin C, Venn C, Walkerdine V (1984) *Changing the Subject*. Methuen, London.
Fanon F (1967) *Black Skin, White Masks*. Grove Press, New York. English Translation by Charles Markmann.
Becker E (1973) *The Denial of Death*. The Free Press, New York.

CHAPTER **TWO**

A challenge to stage theories of dementia

JANET BELL
IAIN McGREGOR

The authors challenge the traditionally-held belief that the progress of dementia follows a predictable and inevitable series of "stages", arguing that this theory inhibits opportunity to explore progressive ways of working with people with dementia.

*T*raditionally, dementia has been seen in simple terms as a progressive, degenerative illness, passing through a series of pre-ordained stages, which inevitably and ultimately end in a terminal vegetative state. We feel that there are serious dangers in adopting this view of dementia, and our experience over the last seven years with people of all ages with dementia has taught us to beware of this simplistic view. Some of the dangers of adopting a stage theory of dementia may be summarised as follows:

• It pre-determines the course of a person's future development, and can thus become a self-fulfilling prophecy.

• It ties each person into a "syndrome", which shifts the emphasis away from the fact that each is a human being with specific identifiable problems.

• It places external limitations on a person's opportunity to realise their true potential.

• It dehumanises the person concerned, so that instead of being regarded as a unique individual, they are seen only in terms of their symptoms.

• It offers a hopeless future of inevitable decline.

• It allows no scope for innovation or progress.

• It lowers the status of the person themselves and of the staff who care for them.

Misconceptions

Over the years, our experience as carers and providers of a resource for people with dementia, (the youngest being only 18 years old), has shown us that there are lots of misconceptions about what dementia does to people, and how they are able to cope with it. The reality is that we are continually surprised by the achievements of our residents, whose determination to succeed in leading normal lives has filled us with a sense of admiration for their dignity and courage (McGregor & Bell 1991).

It has been our observation that people with dementia rarely feel that there is anything wrong with them. They see themselves as normal. In fact if asked whether there is anything about themselves that they would want to change, they will usually appear surprised at the question and reply that they would not want to be any different. It is important therefore that we reconsider our own perception of dementia. We are forced to accept that people with this condition may have potential and possibilities in excess of our pre-conceptions. They have no problem with this themselves.

If we are able to open up *our* minds, perhaps people with dementia may then have the opportunity to extend their own frontiers. It may be that our limited perspectives hold them back from achieving what is possible. We need to liberate our imaginations and then who knows what will happen when we stop limiting their horizons.

As carers, the only generalisation we feel comfortable making about the people with dementia that we have known, is that it primarily affects two areas: memory and communication.

Everyone with dementia has memory problems to some degree or other, some more extensive than others. There are also very commonly difficulties in communication. Most other problems however stem from these two factors, which vary from person to person and whose effects are completely unique to each individual.

In other words, we cannot generalise about dementia, we must always

LOOK AT THE PERSON, NOT THE DIAGNOSIS!

Just because someone loses ability in one or two areas of their functioning, does this mean they become incompetent in every area? Throughout the last seven years we have been able to say with confidence that, without exception, every single person in our care has proved to be a unique individual. Despite the commonly held belief that dementia destroys personality, they have retained the basic core characteristics that made them the person they always were.

Our approach lies in creating a sedative free, supportive environment where residents are enabled to be themselves despite their disability. This allows them to begin to grow, to develop self confidence and a sense of personal worth. Behaviour controlling drugs are jettisoned to be replaced by an environment where the person can start to re-discover their selfhood. Time and again we have witnessed this re-emergence of the old personality, with all its strengths, weaknesses, joys and sadnesses.

Rather than looking upon dementia as a mental disorder, which will follow a series of pre-determined stages, it is more positive and helpful to adopt a similar model to that of the Disability Movement – namely that someone with dementia is a human being, just like the rest of us, but with particular, individual problems. We can and must define these problems specifically, and abandon all generalising statements which put people into categories.

An example of this is the way we use the term *incontinence*. The word itself tells us little about the person or their problem. It is much more helpful to describe exactly which part of the process of going to the toilet is problematic. It may be any one of a number of difficulties: for example, managing their clothing, locating the toilet, communicating the need to go in the first place, and so on. Once we know where the problem lies, the solution is much more obvious, and we can positively set about helping to resolve it.

If, for example, through careful observation we are able to re-define a problem of "incontinence" as "Jim is able to find his way to the toilet unaided, but once he is there he is unable to undo his zip, and therefore wets his trousers", then a number of possible solutions to the problem become apparent. This individualised approach can be used for all the problems we identify.

Similarly the term *paranoia* is commonly used to describe a person's mental state. What in fact usually occurs in dementia however, is that the person concerned is misinterpreting what is happening in their life. Rather than being a psychiatric condition it is more a case of poor memory, insecurity and fear, with the result that the person concerned comes to the only conclusion that makes any sense to them.

Adjusting to disability

As with all disabilities, the individual must adjust in order to experience a positive and fruitful life. People with dementia do this quite naturally. It is however much more difficult for relatives and loved ones, since they are distressed by what is lost, rather than accepting the person as they are now. The most successful caring relationships are those where the person with dementia is accepted just for what they are, not pressurised to become what they once were – an impossible target for them to achieve.

People with dementia experience a strong sense of failure when pushed to function at a level which is no longer possible. The effect of continual exposure to this negative experience is the destruction of self confidence, self image and sense of worth. The person withdraws, stops trying, possibly even living.

The alternative approach of accepting that person just as they are now, while reinforcing their positive qualities and strengths, results in the probability of relationships which were previously damaged being restored. It is the springboard for a rejuvenated relationship.

Anna
Anna was withdrawn, difficult and rejecting. She appeared to have no social aptitude at all, and was a difficult person to relate to. This all changed dramatically however when a new staff member joined the team. He had a genuine affection for Anna, and enjoyed spending time with her, talking to her, laughing and joking. She became relaxed, open and interactive, with the result that the rest of us started to enjoy her company. She displayed skills that had seemed lost for ever, and showed improvement in all areas of her functioning.
(McGregor & Bell 1994a)

As professional carers it is our job to create a "benign social psychology" (Kitwood 1993). Our residents need to believe that they are valued and valuable, loved and appreciated, and that they do have something to offer the rest of us. As they grow in confidence and self-esteem they will start to help others and to accept that they can contribute positively to the group. We ourselves may find it difficult at first to accept that we too have much to learn from people with dementia, and that we can receive as well as give (McGregor & Bell 1994b).

How important is memory?

Memory is obviously essential to our functioning as members of a complex society. In terms of personal value as a human being however, and of our right to a hopeful and positive future, we ought to ask ourselves the following questions:

• Does our personality, and sense of awareness of ourselves as unique and individual human beings depend upon having a good memory?

• Without a good memory:
  – can we be a fulfilled human being?
  – are we less valuable as a human being?
  – have we nothing positive to offer "normal" society?

Memory is the depository of many aspects of our daily lives. Apart from facts, we remember such things as ideas, friendship, love, likes and dislikes, good and bad. Dementia does not destroy these. People still remember love; they are still able to express and experience love, and to form new and lasting relationships. The basic personhood of someone with dementia – their feelings, emotions and responses – remains intact long after they have ceased to be able to communicate in language.

Personality is clearly influenced by a person's unique adjustment to their environment. In residential or nursing care however, we are the architects who create that environment, therefore becoming responsible to our residents for offering opportunities that will enable them to regain their sense of selfhood and personality. We will have to demonstrate imagination and innovation, and approach the task with a completely open mind.

Charter of rights

It is important to establish some fundamental principles on which to base our work with dementia. At Spring Mount we have formulated the following charter of rights:

We believe that any person with dementia:
• has equal value as a human being to anyone else
• will function better both intellectually and physically without the use of tranquillising drugs
• always retains some degree of insight
• has the same rights to the highest quality of life as anyone else
• always retains some ability for new learning even though the process may take longer
• is capable of developing and enjoying social relationships and friendships
• retains his or her basic personality
• always possesses the potential to be a valued human being
• knows when he or she is happy and content.
(McGregor & Bell 1993)

Stage theories of dementia predict an inevitable outlook. They assert that the illness slowly and irretrievably destroys personality, that patients lose insight, and become unaware of their surroundings. Even with people in a coma we are rightly very careful to maintain the principle that they are able to understand what is happening around them, that they understand what is being said about them and that they have insight into their situation. It seems that we are not prepared to make this same commitment to people with dementia, which may consequently only serve to justify provision of the worst resources and treatment.

On the other hand if the environment is helpful and constructive, a person with dementia can begin the process of re-discovering and rebuilding aspects of themselves that were previously stifled by inhibition and social conditioning.

People with dementia naturally adjust to the changes that occur to themselves and their lives. In this sense they are no different to the rest of us. We all have to adjust to change, growing old, infirmity and so on. Provided we do not interfere with this process, and allow it to take its natural course, they will be able to navigate their way through life with their self image intact. Like the rest of us they need to be free of the constant battle to avoid the threat of annihilation of the self. They need to feel valued and valuable, self-accepting and self confident.

Frances
Frances was always very concerned about her appearance. She is described as having been conscientiously smart and tidy. Now she wears three dresses, two cardigans and a pair of trousers underneath. Does this mean that her basic personality has changed? She is still the same kind, loving, gentle person she always was. She is never aggressive, still very sociable, with a ready wisecrack. She is, in fact, still extremely concerned about her appearance. What she has lost is the discernment to know what is socially acceptable dressing. In her opinion she is smart. Frances is still a strong-willed, independent individual, which makes it difficult to influence her choice of clothing. (McGregor & Bell 1994c)

It is essential for people with dementia that we respect their diverse, idiosyncratic and elaborate ways of experiencing their personal sense of existence, even though this may be at odds with our preconceptions. This will then become a source of creativity, and will allow them to embark on their own personal voyage of discovery.

It seems to us who are privileged to partake in so many people's voyages, that a stage theory of dementia is not only irrelevant but positively dangerous.

References
Kitwood T (1993) Person and process in dementia. *International Journal of Geriatric Psychiatry* **8(7)** 541-546.
McGregor I, Bell J (1991) Living for the moment. *Nursing Times* **87(18)** 45-47.
McGregor I, Bell J (1993) Voyage of discovery. *Nursing Times* **89(36)** 29-31.
McGregor I, Bell J (1994a) Beyond the mask of conventional manners. *Journal of Dementia Care* **2(5)** 18-19.
McGregor I, Bell J (1994b) Buzzing with life, energy and drive. *Journal of Dementia Care* **2(6)** 20-21.
McGregor I, Bell J (1994c) Breaking free from myths that restrain us. *Journal of Dementia Care* **2(4)** 14-15.

CHAPTER THREE

Sharing the care: towards new forms of communication

JEAN TOBIN

Family carers look for some relief and support from professionals, but they would like to be recognised as partners in an enterprise of shared care, whether from a family base or in long-term care settings. The way this principle could work in practice, and lead to more satisfactory care from all points of view, is discussed.

People who choose to care for their dementing relatives do so from a background of lifelong mutual support. They generally bring to the task commitment, love and a positive attitude, at least at the beginning. Committed carers share a history and some characteristics with their relatives and these are advantages in their efforts to care successfully.

In this chapter I consider three main issues – what a carer is, shared care from a family base, and shared care in long-term settings. The views expressed here are mine, but I believe they reflect those of family carers who want to care for their dementing relative, and whose circumstances allow them to do so. To avoid tedium, and, as the majority of family carers and people with dementia are female, I use only the feminine gender when referring to either group.

Shared experience

For the family carer, the person they care for is a parent or partner first and foremost, not an old confused person with whom it is difficult to make contact. Interests and hobbies are known and can be kept alive in some form for as long as possible. Reassurance can be based on shared experience, and present happenings can be related to those in the past and the future. Also family carers surely have a better chance than anyone of understanding "problem behaviour", and responding to the underlying unmet need which such behaviour reveals. For all these reasons carers believe that, in most instances, the highest quality of life for a dementing person is to be found in their family and that is why we strive so hard to provide family care. However, as the dementia progresses, it becomes harder for one or two people to care for 24 hours a day, seven days a week. So we look for relief and support.

Carers have woken up to the fact that much dementia care has been of a very low standard. We believe that something better is needed and is possible today. We

have what we regard as reasonable expectations of civilised care.

After all, we have left the age of the asylum when people with dementia were locked away from the community and care was only of a basic physical kind. Then the very limited medical model of dementia held sway, offering no guidelines or hope for care. The ignorance of relatives and the general public, and the mystique of the medical profession, allowed this to happen. We now live in an age when education is concerned with understanding, not learning by rote, when Psychology and English Literature are two of the most popular subjects read at university – subjects concerned with human life, its motivations and relationships.

Many documentaries on TV present us with the lives of all sorts and conditions of men (and women) and how they can survive in adverse circumstances through the indomitability of the human spirit and the help of loving, caring and resourceful people. So it makes sense if professional carers adopt a similar positive attitude. Family carers want their dementing relatives to be treated as we ourselves would like to be treated. Nothing less is good enough.

A few family carers live in places where good quality dementia care is available from social services, but still in many areas, much of the support and relief they need is non-existent or patchy or uncoordinated or of poor quality. They are no longer prepared to put up with people working in dementia care who do not know what they are doing. So family carers may get angry as they try to assert their rights and needs, on behalf of their relative. They may appear arrogant in doing so, which is something they often accuse professionals of being! However, we believe that family and paid carers must value and appreciate each other's skills and work together for the benefit of dementing people.

What is a carer?

Let us look at some of the findings (Fig 1) of one research project, "Caring for carers", which is nearing completion after four years work (Logan 1994).

No one will be surprised by the huge difference in hours per week spent caring by family and paid carers. It is probably the main reason for the exhaustion of family carers. So it is remarkable to discover that they manage to continue the task for five years – surely a

FAMILY carers provide care for an average of 100 hours per week.	PAID carers provide care for an average of 31 hours per week.
FAMILY carers' overall average duration of caregiving is 5 years.	PAID carers' overall average duration of caregiving is 3 years.
FAMILY carers' relatives are almost as severely impaired and show more socially disturbed behaviour.	PAID carers look after residents who are more disabled in terms of physical disability, apathy and communication difficulties.
FAMILY carers reported higher levels of distress and dissatisfaction.	PAID carers reported higher levels of life satisfaction.

FAMILY and PAID carers both exceed average scores, obtained from similar community samples, on psychological distress and poorer life satisfaction.

Figure 1. Findings of the Caring for Carers Project

measure of their resolve and commitment. The equivalent three year average figure for paid carers is worrying because it implies a lack of continuity of care for patients, which makes good quality care less likely. Turnover may be due to poor working conditions (pay, consideration, status, training) all of which probably means that they are undervalued as persons in their own right and as caregivers.

The next two statements show that there is little difference between the disabilities of dementing people in a care home and those still at home. Perhaps the latter show more socially disturbed behaviour because they have not given up fighting for their needs, not yet become apathetic. Conversely, those who have moved to a care home may have been set free from a poor family relationship.

The different levels of satisfaction of family and paid carers are not surprising. One would not expect a high level of life satisfaction if one is working over 100 hours per week alone, and at such a difficult and demanding task. The last finding confirms this, for it suggests that giving care to a person with dementia is a more distressing occupation than caring for other patient groups, and particularly so when that care is provided in the family.

Another finding from the project is that certain family carers are more vulnerable to stress because of their personality, which affects their perception of their caring situation and the coping style they adopt. An extravert personality will pick up the phone and ask for help while a neurotic anxious carer will be afraid to do this. (What the author of this work does not consider is

the personality of the dementing person. We think this is a crucial factor affecting the ability of family carers to cope and the level of stress they feel).

The findings discussed here confirm much that we already suspected. The insights are based on sound and comprehensive research and show a real concern for family carers.

Reclassifying the carer

The annual expenditure on dementia by mental health services alone has been estimated at £189m. Much of the burden of care falls on informal carers who contribute an estimated £11,600m worth of care per year. (North Thames Regional Health Authority 1994).

It seems incredible that family carers are still being called "informal" carers, when research tells us that they work about 100 hours a week, and common sense tells us they are on call for the whole 168 hours in every week.

Let us make a distinction based on the way a person with dementia is cared for, instead of where that care occurs. I will use "real" and "formal" as the labels, and define them in a relevant way:

Real carers see people with dementia as human beings first and foremost. They see the likeness to themselves, the common humanity, but they also respond to the individual. **Formal carers** have a more detached or uninvolved approach. They see the disability first, not the person, and they treat all dementia sufferers in a similar way as they make no attempt to learn about them.

Shared care from a family base

We believe that real carers, both family and paid, should cooperate and share care throughout a dementing person's life, wherever that care takes place. So when family carers look for help and relief from paid carers, this would not mean that the care was taken out of their hands completely. Let us examine how this could work in practice as we follow the typical caring route.

Family carers hope to care at home for as long as possible – in fact they have the sincere intention, at the beginning, to care until the end of their relatives' lives. Above all, they need informed support from all the community services – GPs, dentists, district nurses, occupational therapists, community psychiatric nurses and so on – all the paramedics with whom a dementing person living at home may be involved.

Why is it that when a person with chronic physical disabilities is discharged from hospital, ramps, hoists, and district nurses appear at their home far more readily than for the person with dementia, who lives at home but also needs help to remain there? Somehow the same rules do not seem to apply.

I heard a senior doctor, a specialist in incontinence, suggest, at a conference, that family carers could fit catheters at home for their relative, and we know of cases when they have been required to insert suppositories and enemas. Do these people believe that dementing people are not their responsibility but should be in the hands of the mental health services? Family carers are fed up with being victims of buck-passing. Or is it that, as they can see no actual disability, they really don't understand the problems that family carers face?

All doctors need to become more informed about dementia. The GP is usually the first influential professional to whom a carer goes with their relative. They may receive a faulty diagnosis or a brutal one and leave in despair with no information, help or advice.

Hospital visits

Doctors and nurses should be aware also of the strain they inflict on dementing people and their carers when they expect the dementia sufferer to be ready and waiting to be examined or bathed at home, or to wait indefinitely for attention in the surgery, hospital or X-ray queue.

Requests for some priority from receptionists or ward clerks are met with blank incomprehension. More domiciliary visits are the answer, but here again we have the situation where there is a ready acceptance of home visits for the physically disabled, but not for the person with dementia. Surgery and hospital visits can be an ordeal for family carers, taxing their patience, skill and resolve to the limit. The message is that most dementia sufferers cannot be expected to sit patiently and wait!

Day care

The quality of day care is enormously variable and so is a dementing person's response to even the best of it. Some people seem to enjoy going out for a day "to meet their friends" or "go to work", and for them day care is a happy experience, but for others it is unsettling. "Where am I going? Why do I have to go?" Waiting for transport or enduring a long, bumpy journey can cause anxiety and distress for the rest of the day. The dementing person returns home between three and five o'clock, often in a bad state physically and mentally. Family carers are left to pick up the pieces and wonder if the short break was worth the effort.

Care at home

Much better in every way is a care attendant coming to the house for two or three hours once or twice a week. This individual care is less hassle and usually more successful. A new development on these lines involves the person with dementia spending two days a week, or so, with another family nearby.

There is another way in which domiciliary care could be supplied and which has always existed for those who have the money to pay. A carer pays one or two people to help her, much like a nanny or *au pair* is used by a mother of young children.

The advantages are that many different people are not coming and going at all hours; the dementing person does not have to leave her own home; and the organisation can be completely in the hands of the carer and so adapted to suit her needs and the sufferer's. One objection might be that skilled people are needed – but family carers usually have no training and learn from experience. Many of them would happily engage a local person with caring skills learned practically in their own family, and find someone whose personality, manner and style suited them and their relative.

Payment to a carer for such a purpose could be made by social services with some of the money saved from providing the services themselves. No mother or family carer would expect to reduce her load to a 40-hour week like a normal job, but she could employ someone to help *her* for 40 hours a week, at a cost of about £160. This is much cheaper than the cost of services supplied to some family carers now, and far less than the fees for residential or nursing homes. Last year Bradford social services provided domiciliary help to one family carer at a cost of £600 per week (Bradford social services 1993). The London borough of Westminster has a ceiling of £500 (Butterworth 1994).

In the *au pair* model, the care package and its management is firmly in the hands of the family carer. She organises things to suit her needs. If she were able to do this in the present set-up, she could choose from the services available so provision would be fitted to the family rather than the other way round.

A neighbourhood centre for dementia care?

Those family carers whose relatives respond well to day care would prefer it to be much more flexible, which is possible when such care is provided in a home or centre which is open all hours. Then people would attend at times to suit themselves and their carers. Also this day care could expand into an occasional overnight stay, a weekend and finally a week's stay so that respite care was being provided in the same place. The family would have to get to know only one institution and its staff – instead of the three or more that are often used now for different types of care. Staff too would know their families much better.

A neighbourhood Dementia Centre like this would welcome shared care so that family carers could help there when they wished. The alternatives to day care – like individual home care by a care attendant – two or three times a week – could be used if preferred – and the complementary night sitting service also. When needs changed, as they do, as needs are never static, it should be possible for the family carer to make different arrangements, perhaps increasing or decreasing some types of service, or substituting an alternative.

Shared care in long-term settings

There are several reasons why long-term care has left a lot to be desired and therefore made it hard for family carers to accept it. The first reason is that it is usually an abrupt transition instead of a gradual change. (This was illustrated for me by the shock of an old man who one day was caring for his wife at home, and the next was a visitor in a long stay unit). Second, the long-term placement has meant abandonment of all responsibility for day-to-day care by the family carer (shared care would solve this). Third, it has been assumed that the situation will not be reversed, that the dementing person will never return home again. Finally, and most importantly, the quality of the care has not been acceptable. (To improve it, some staff may have to be re-trained before they can provide what is needed.)

We want care to be person-centred – that is care "which focuses on relationship, on communication, on individuality, and on the feelings and abilities that are retained" by a dementing person (Kitwood & Bredin 1992). We want relatives to be welcomed and encouraged to share that caregiving with the staff, instead of being regarded as a threat or a nuisance. We want staff to understand our wish to continue to take part in the care of our relative: to understand that for us to be able to go home for a good sleep, and return refreshed the next day to help again, would be no great hardship. And similarly, to realise that when one has struggled at home with every aspect of care for years, to feed one's relative with good food, cooked and brought to you by others, is bliss.

Gradually some of us may come in less frequently, or stay for less time, but we would like shared care to be accepted in long-term care as well as in the community, so that those carers who wish to participate may do so. The family carer would be included in the making of care plans for their relative, and in the regular review with the GP and the staff at the care home or centre.

A long-term place in an already known and trusted Dementia Centre, where shared care was the norm, would make the decision to give up caring at home much easier. It could be easier, too, for the patient to return home if circumstances changed, so that the decision to place someone in long term care was not considered irrevocable.

Rights and risk

We believe people with dementia are at risk in many homes because insufficient precautions are taken to avoid accidents. The reasons for this come from muddled thinking about "infantilisation", "rights", "freedom" and "liberty" and the acceptance of generalisations about the abilities of people with dementia. Risk-taking is considered acceptable, so there are many accidents, some of which lead directly or indirectly to death. *Home Life: a Code of Practice for Residential Care* (DHSS 1984) refers to "responsible risk-taking", and the word "responsible" makes a great difference. Some risk would be acceptable if all reasonable precautions, all sensible steps, had been taken, but this is not always the case. As for "infantilisation", if one can wash, pad and feed without it, surely with forethought and supervision, one can protect from danger without it too.

What carers expect

To summarise:
• We would like community services to be more informed about dementia so that they can offer us better support.
• We would like flexible day care to be offered alongside night care and respite care in a community Dementia Centre, which could also provide long-term places.
• We would like the family carer to be able to choose from the community services available and to take charge of his/her relative's care package.
• We want long-term care to be of a good quality, to come about through a gradual transition, and to be easily reversible.
• Finally and most importantly, we want to share, with real paid carers, the delivery of dementia care, wherever and whenever it takes place. We believe this would benefit the three groups involved in the process, and it makes sense to use family carers' skills for as long as they are prepared to offer them.

We believe that good dementia care is built on the essential requirement of all good relationships, which is to take the other person, in this case the person with dementia, as seriously as we take ourselves. This basic principle needs to be applied to family carers too, and if it is, the new culture of dementia care will include genuine partnership and cooperation.

References
Logan C (1994) *Caregiving to older people who have a dementia: coping, individual differences and the context of care.* DPhil thesis, University of Oxford.
North Thames Regional Health Authority (1994) *Research and Development Programme in Mental Health.*
Assistant Director of Social Services, Bradford (1993).
Butterworth M (1994) Personal communication.
Kitwood T and Bredin K (1992) *Person to Person.* Gale Centre Publications, Loughton, Essex.
DHSS/Centre for Policy on Ageing (1984) *Home Life: a Code of Practice for Residential Care.*

The beginnings of a new culture in care

CHAPTER FOUR

BOB WOODS

The new culture has roots in numerous attempts to recognise the human value, worth and potential of people with dementia. Similar developments are apparent in related fields, such as that of learning difficulties. Achieving the new culture requires changes at all levels; staff support is essential.

*T*he new culture of dementia care represents a dramatic change in philosophy, attitudes and practice. The identification of aspects of care that must change is not difficult: the devaluation, invalidation and dehumanisation of people with dementia has often been described; the environments where care is provided have often left much to be desired (Woods & Britton 1985). The new culture, on the other hand, is characterised by:

• its emphasis on **values**; it values the person with dementia as a full human being and does not perceive him/her as an object or a sub-human life-form.

• its recognition of the role of the **environment**; the person with cognitive impairment is perhaps more dependent on his/her immediate environment (physical and social) than most people, and less able than most to take steps, unaided, to adjust, adapt and control all aspects of it.

• the **individualisation** of care; each person with dementia is recognised as an individual, with a unique set of life experiences, preferences, values, abilities and needs, which must be understood in getting to know the **whole person.**

• efforts to achieve effective two-way **communication**; the onus is on the care-giver to find ways of improving their own communication skills, verbal and non-verbal, and to become a better listener, rather than simply bemoaning the person with dementia's impairment.

These ideas, however, are of course by no means completely new, and efforts to implement some of these features can be traced back for many years. In addition, other areas of care provision – such as that for people with learning difficulties – have gone through a process of change showing some similar directions. This chapter aims firstly to describe the roots of the new culture in the dementia care field, before making the comparison with parallel changes in the care of people with learning difficulties. Finally, areas which the new culture will have to address if it is to become a lasting reality will be identified.

The roots of good dementia care

We do not then need to start completely from scratch in creating a new culture; there have in fact been many examples over the years of attempts to implement dementia care in a way that recognises the human value and worth of the person. What has been lacking has been a culture where such approaches have been widely accepted and implemented in a manner sensitive to the person with dementia's individual needs. There is still much to be learned from these efforts, which may be viewed as the early roots of the new culture. Among them could be included:

Activity and stimulation

These approaches, which may be traced back at least 35 years (Holden & Woods 1988), were clearly based on the notion that people with dementia were capable of responding to their surroundings, and that enriching their environment was a worthwhile endeavour.

Some workers thought of the person with dementia as being deprived of sensory and social input, and sought to redress this through increased stimulation. Music, exercise, activity of various kinds were offered. At times the approach has been over-zealous and not sufficiently sensitive to individual preferences, but at its core is an awareness of the under-functioning of many people with dementia, arising from the impoverished, unstimulating environments in which they spend their time.

Reality orientation (RO)

This approach, much maligned of late, has its roots in the USA, also over 30 years ago, where again there was recognition of greater potential for response in the person with dementia than had previously been envisaged. The aim was to give direct care staff a positive way of interacting, focusing particularly on the disorientation so often encountered in dementia.

A large body of research has subsequently evaluated changes in orientation and behavioural function; it is, though, interesting that among the changes noted by the American pioneers of this approach were that patients' "look of hopelessness changed to hopefulness" when they began RO (Holden & Woods 1988).

This early insight into the well-being of people with dementia was unfortunately swamped by a caricature of the approach being applied in many locations, where confrontation was used unhelpfully, and information given without thought to individual needs. I have argued elsewhere that there remain many lessons to be learned from the RO literature (Woods 1992), not least that learning potential is not completely lost in dementia, and that an individualised approach is vital.

Reminiscence

Reminiscence work with older people with dementia was given a major impetus with the availability of the Help the Aged *Recall* tape-slide packs in the early 1980s. These were designed to trigger memories from the then current generation of older people's earlier years, using photographs, music and archive sound material depicting everyday life as well as those historical events that impinged on most people's lives.

Again there was the very positive aim of bringing more response from the person with dementia than was normally the case; drawing on the person's store of long-term memories, which often appeared better preserved than those more recently experienced; through a more biographical approach (Gibson 1994) allowing staff and other carers to get to know the person more fully as a whole person, in the context of a life-span of experience, relationships and achievements.

Validation therapy

Validation therapy was developed by Naomi Feil (1993) partly in response to dissatisfaction with RO, with its emphasis on "correct" information, and at times an apparent lack of empathy for the perspective of the person with dementia.

Validation encourages the worker to communicate on a deeper level, by drawing attention to the emotional content, rather than remaining on the surface level of "facts". It aims to restore dignity and prevent decline into a withdrawn state, through the contact with an empathic listener who does not judge the person's view of reality, but offers acceptance and respect. Its aims and methods fit fairly readily with the new culture, although it might be said to perhaps over-emphasise the role of unresolved conflicts from the past as underlying the emotions communicated.

Stokes and Goudie (1990) describe *resolution therapy*, which also encourages reflective, empathic listening, and similarly draws attention to the emotional content of the person with dementia's efforts to communicate. They similarly argue that behind what the person says or does there may be a "concealed meaning".

In resolution therapy there is greater awareness that this may relate to a current concern, rather than assuming an unresolved conflict from the past to be always present.

Both approaches then have recognised the importance of valuing and respecting the person as an individual, of developing communication. Resolution therapy has given greater attention to the impact of the current environment on behaviour and interaction, but both approaches are based on the principle that the way in which people interact with the person with dementia now can make an appreciable difference to his or her well-being. Neither approach has yet attracted much in the way of systematic empirical evaluation.

Special care units

There has been a recent trend towards residential units specialising in the individualised care of people with dementia in homely, domestic settings, which all share the implicit assumption that the person's surroundings and the regime of care make a considerable difference to the person's quality of life. The person is to receive not just physical care, but care that recognises the diversity of their needs. In Britain there have been "domus" units, in France "cantou" (a word for hearth), in Sweden group-living homes and "integrity-promoting care". Not all have shaken off entirely the vestiges of the institution, but in many a real effort has been made to develop a better quality of life (Holden & Woods 1995).

Support for families

While some doubt the motives of the increasing support for families of people with dementia, fearing it is primarily a cost-saving exercise, there is no doubt that much good work has been done in this area (Moriarty & Levin 1993). If it is recognised that many older people with dementia would prefer care at home, by those known to them, the value of this approach in preserving some important aspects of life for the dementia sufferer is clear. If the family carer is enabled to experience less strain, then the person with dementia's quality of life is also likely to improve. As is well known, this approach too may break down: abuse, difficult relationships, neglect and dehumanisation may occur in the family setting, just as in the institution.

What can we learn from other fields?

It can be useful at times to look beyond the confines of dementia care, to examine how the care of other groups with disabilities is developing. For example, many of the concerns regarding the effects of institutions on people with dementia over the years have been exactly paralleled in services for people with learning difficulties and those with severe mental illness. Here will be discussed some of the recurrent themes arising from the learning difficulties field, in order to place dementia care in a broader perspective.

Behaviour modification has been a major force, reflecting the emergence of the notion that learning and development are possible, under the right conditions. This has helped to prevent people with learning difficulties being written off completely. It is probably mirrored in dementia care by approaches such as RO.

Normalisation, a theory of how and why people with disabilities are devalued through labelling, inappropriate images and so on, is applicable across all disabilities (including dementia), but has been most influential in the learning difficulties field, where it led to the concept of **ordinary living** – people with learning difficulties living in ordinary houses, not set apart from the rest of the community, as had been the case in the big, institutional hospitals they replaced.

Concerns about misconceptions of normalisation, which seemed to lay emphasis on making people "normal' (whatever that may be!) have led to it being re-named **social role valorisation**, with a definition that emphasises the encouragement of roles, experiences and behaviour that are valued in society. The person's dignity, choice, individuality, independence and social relationships are encouraged. These principles are most clearly seen applied to dementia care in the Kings Fund paper *Living well into old age* (1986).

No approach can ignore the special needs of the client group, and in the learning difficulties field much attention has been given to **"challenging behaviour"** (formerly known as behaviour problems). Special units and teams have been established, and the change in name reflects a genuine concern not to see the problem as residing in the person with learning difficulties, but as a real challenge to all involved to find a way forward. Individual programme plans, often developed from behaviour modification principles, have been the major strategy, apart from medication, in tackling challenging behaviour.

Recently, there has been interest in, and controversy around, an alternative approach, **gentle teaching** (Jones and Connell 1993). This places greater emphasis on the attitude of the care-giver and on human engagement with the person. The approach is concerned with the whole person, mind, body, emotions and spirit, not just observable behaviour. The client is valued unconditionally, and the care-giver does not "modify" the client, but rather seeks mutual change.

The movement towards greater human engagement at an emotional level is illustrated by the growth of the use of **psychotherapy** with people with learning difficulties. A similar trend may be noted in dementia care (Hausman 1992, Sinason 1992).

Clearly then, in the field of learning difficulties, approaches which more fully reflect the personhood of the client are gaining ground, and there are many parallels with dementia care. One may argue that the new culture of dementia care reflects broader changes in our understanding of society's devaluing response to disability, as well as specific insights regarding the nature of dementia.

Making it happen

The story so far of high quality dementia care is one of good intentions, but little consistent, long-term change. Too often, therapeutic programmes have become a travesty of the original, or have been abandoned prematurely. It is suggested that achieving a new culture in the real world will be aided by considering the following issues:

Involve families

Professional care-givers have a complex relationship with relatives/family carers of dementia sufferers. In the community, they are the key to the person with dementia remaining in his/her home. Their sense of strain has been extensively documented, and at times leads to uncertainty as to who is the professional's client – the person with dementia or the carer.

The different perspective the family carer has on the person with dementia, after perhaps many years together, combined with the strain-related fragility of the situation, leads to sensitive professionals being reluctant to intervene too strongly, so as to not upset the delicate existing balance.

Yet if the new culture is to have an impact in the community, families have to be full partners in this enterprise. Day-centres and sitting services can doubtless make a difference, but it is with family members that many people with dementia spend most of their time. Involving family carers in, say, reminiscence or RO approaches at home has not proved easy, and considerable thought must be given as to how they may be helped to take their place in the new culture.

In the residential setting, the other side of the coin is seen. How often staff complain that the relatives are more trouble than the residents! Family carers can often see aspects of the care they would like to be improved, although rarely do they have a place where this can be expressed safely and securely. Complaints may be written off as reflecting relatives' guilt, although more often relatives keep quiet for fear of repercussions affecting their loved one.

Forging a partnership between relatives/family carers and professionals has proved difficult both in the community and in residential settings. The new culture requires the contribution and perspective of family members to be valued and worked with, not to be by-passed or marginalised.

Staff morale and job satisfaction

The new culture is demanding of staff; it asks for increased human, personal engagement with the person with dementia, which can be draining and taxing. Burn-out is an issue that must be addressed. It may be recognised in feelings of emotional exhaustion, negative attitudes towards those for whom one is providing care, perhaps depersonalisation, not seeing "them" as people, a feeling of dissatisfaction with what is accomplished in the job and a tendency to evaluate one's work performance negatively.

There are many factors which have been shown to contribute to burn-out. Some are specific to the person – their ways of coping, their general psychological resilience; others relate more to the context of work. Although some recent studies suggest that those providing care for people with dementia are no more emotionally distressed than the general population, there is no doubt that the new culture will place greatly increased emotional demands on staff, and will challenge the familiar defence of maintaining a distance between oneself and the person with dementia. The new culture must therefore be accompanied by greatly increased support for staff, valuing their skills and contribution, and recognising the issues raised by daily confronting loss of skills and abilities, and by frequent exposure to death.

Structure and policies

It is not enough for staff providing direct care to embrace the new culture. Those responsible for managing the service must be fully behind the staff, if they are to receive the support and enabling required. This goes beyond rhetoric, the stated policies of the service; the question must be what is actually encouraged by the management – do they really value good dementia care?

As ever, actions speak louder than words in this sphere. Are staff given the time and resources to provide personal care? Are promotions within the service related to quality of care? Is there a clarity of structure, avoiding ambiguity about decision making? Do staff have a say in how the service is run? Are their views taken seriously?

These issues may perhaps be summarised as reflecting the extent to which staff themselves are valued by the organisation. If they do not themselves feel valued, will it not be more difficult for them to value those for whom they provide care? This principle is embodied as one of the four tenets of the philosophy underlying the "domus" special care units (Lindesay et al 1991), which states that the needs of staff should be considered equally with those of the residents.

Some may feel a resistance to such a statement,

fearing a return to a culture where the home or ward was apparently run very much for the convenience and ease of the staff, and where residents were stripped of dignity and individuality. This reflected a gross power imbalance, where staff abused the enormous power they had over people's day-to-day lives. Equal consideration for staff and residents, on the other hand, reflects a balanced approach, where no group is to be down-graded and devalued.

Adequate resources are clearly needed for staff to feel valued and supported, and for there to be sufficient staff to provide individualised care. However, resources alone are not enough; there needs to be clarity of communication and an effective use of resources to achieve the desired quality of care. More staff is not the answer if the extra staff are, for example, reinforcing dependence or interacting in an unhelpful manner. Those in management positions have a crucial role to play if the new culture is to become a reality.

Quality assurance or quality control?

With a history of abortive attempts to change the care environment for people with dementia, the issue arises as to how the new culture can be maintained. Can it become self-driven, with a group of staff monitoring their own progress, or is a perspective from outside required?

For example, in the USA an effective way of reducing levels of incontinence has been developed (prompted voiding), which should benefit patients and staff (Schnelle et al 1993). It requires a little extra input from staff, but should be well worthwhile as it demonstrably reduces the times a patient has to be changed out of wet clothing. However, in implementation after implementation of this approach, staff stopped carrying out the required procedures almost as soon as the demonstration project has ended. The project workers have now developed a "quality control" procedure, which involves regular checks on practice, and have shown that this maintained the programme much better than general exhortations and demonstrations.

The new culture of dementia care is too important, we could argue, to leave to staff to monitor themselves through the usual quality assurance procedures. It will also require quality control, systematic and regular checks on performance, if it is to become an enduring feature of dementia care.

Research-based approach

There will, then, be many obstacles placed in the way of the new culture of dementia care, many barriers to progress, many reasons why old ways may not be changed. There is a great deal to be done before the pockets of good practice come together to form the new culture.

There remains a dearth of good quality research on these aspects of dementia care, despite the current climate in the health and social services encouraging a research-based approach to changing practice. Evidence needs to be marshalled indicating the difference that can be made to the quality of life of the person with dementia. This will require more sensitive measures of the well-being of the person with dementia; clearer empirical descriptions of the web of interactions around the person; and systematic observations and record-keeping to document the improvements and stability in cases of dementia that defy the text-book definitions, but which have been recounted by many in the field.

Families and skilled practitioners must join with researchers in this endeavour, which must go beyond the small-scale work that has been the norm in the past. Funding bodies must recognise that while research is of course necessary on the biological aspects of dementia and on possible pharmacological therapies, improving the quality of dementia care also merits some priority in funding.

Whatever the biological and pharmacological breakthroughs, it is absolutely clear that dementia care will continue to be a major concern for our society for many years to come. Achieving and maintaining the new culture remains vital; all the indications are that the movement is well under way.

References

Feil N (1993) *The Validation breakthrough: simple techniques for communicating with people with "Alzheimer's type dementia"*. Health Professions Press, Baltimore.

Gibson F (1994) What can reminiscence contribute to people with dementia? In Bornat J (Ed), *Reminiscence reviewed: evaluations, achievements, perspectives*. Open University Press, Buckingham. pp46 – 60.

Hausman C, (1992) Dynamic psychotherapy with elderly demented patients. In Jones G, Miesen BML (Eds) *Care-giving in dementia: research and applications*. Routledge, London. pp181-198.

Holden UP, Woods RT (1988) *Reality orientation: psychological approaches to the "confused" elderly* (Second edition). Churchill Livingstone, Edinburgh.

Holden UP, Woods RT (1995) *Positive approaches to dementia care*. Churchill Livingstone, Edinburgh.

Jones RSP, Connell E, (1993) Ten years of gentle teaching: much ado about nothing? *The Psychologist*, **6 (12)** 544-548.

King's Fund (1986) *Living well into old age: applying principles of good practice to services for elderly people with severe mental disabilities*. King's Fund, London.

Lindesay J, Briggs K, Lawes M, Macdonald A, Herzberg J (1991) The domus philosophy: a comparative evaluation of a new approach to residential care for the demented elderly. *International Journal of Geriatric Psychiatry* **6** 727-736.

Moriarty J, Levin E (1993) Interventions to assist caregivers. *Reviews in Clinical Gerontology*, **3** 301-308.

Schnelle JF, Newman D, White M, Abbey J, Wallston KA, Fogarty T, Ory MG (1993) Maintaining continence in nursing home residents through the application of industrial quality control. *Gerontologist* **33** 114-121.

Sinason V (1992) The man who was losing his brain. In Sinason V (Ed) *Mental handicap and the human condition: new approaches from the Tavistock*. Free Association Books, London. pp87-110.

Stoke G, Goudie F (1990) Counselling confused elderly people. In Stokes G, Goudie F (Eds) *Working with dementia*. Winslow Press, Bicester. pp181-190.

Woods RT, Britton PG (1985) *Clinical psychology with the elderly*. Croom Helm/Chapman Hall, London, chapter 9.

Woods RT (1992) What can be learned from studies on reality orientation? In Jones G, Miesen BML (Eds) *Care-giving in dementia*. Routledge, London. pp121 – 136.

Holden UP, Woods RT (1988) *Reality orientation: psychological approaches to the "confused" elderly* (Second edition). Churchill Livingstone, Edinburgh.

CHAPTER FIVE | People with dementia can communicate – if we are able to hear

BRIGITTE A FRANK

The research described here affirms that people with dementia can and do communicate. In a care culture that values the interpersonal context, conversations can unfold, emotions are expressed, relationships develop. Competence in communication, so often overlooked or denied, needs to be valued and nurtured.

*I*t is frequently thought that those who have dementia are unable to communicate appropriately, either with their carers or with each other, and that much of their conversation is doomed to be meaningless. Drastic though this view may sound, it is not entirely fictional (Bohling 1991). It is also true that one of the hallmarks of life in a nursing home has been identified as "forlorn silence" (Kaakinen 1992). This chapter attempts to sketch aspects of communicative interaction among elderly people with dementia in a nursing home, where the emphasis is on person-centred care (Kitwood 1993).

My intention was to make a bold claim and to gather some evidence for it: people with dementia have something to say and they do say it; they do more than just respond or soliloquise – despite the impact of whatever neuropathology there may be in their brains.

My account is based on a series of dementia care mapping (DCM) evaluations (Kitwood & Bredin 1992; see also chapter 15) and a relatively small sample of audio-recorded episodes of everyday spoken conversations, collected between December 1993 and March 1994.

My ambition was certainly not to trivialise any carer's (or resident's) stress and frustrations; nor, indeed, to create a revolutionary theory of human communication. Rather, I hope to redress the balance somewhat by trying to associate dementia with "competence". This is a connection often shunned rather than discovered. Competence can be re-discovered, affirmed, and positively considered in relation to "performance" among peers. This competence is so easily belittled or overlooked – if not denied – where we expect only deficits. My aim, then, was to carry out research **with** people rather than **on** them; person-centred care has its counterpart in person-centred research.

Any type of social interaction will have immediate consequences for morale, psychological well-being and therefore health. Looking at conversation, however fragmented and contradictory, as a developing process rather than a finished product, our aim must include highlighting participants' achievements rather than merely their deficits. Caring observation concerned with whole persons may yield some insight into the quality of life in terms of talk.

Research background

Clinical research in the field has yielded invaluable insights about the nature and presenting features of dementing disorders, and (to a lesser degree) about forms of interventions; the merits of such work are known and deserve to be widely acknowledged.

At the same time, a vast body of relevant literature emphasises a dissolution of cognition in dementia (Lee 1991). Divorced from the clinical context for which it was originally designed, it appears to authorise a view of communication as advancing conversational anarchy. Confronted with batteries of tests, elements of which would baffle people with no neurological impairments, the "assessed-to-be" readily commit errors of colourful description: they fluently introduce themselves in all vagueness; insensitively abandon utterances; persevere in nonsensical responses. Besides, nobody may be all that clear as to who or what is being referred to, and instead end up less intelligible and more confused than ever.

Language, especially spoken language, can reveal (and conceal) much about a person. Linguistic pathologies in particular are immediately noticeable, even more so than physical impairments; therefore, they lead more readily to stigmatizations. (Mis-)led to see the "patients" as embodiments of abnormal conditions, our starting point for meaningful interactions does not afford much hope. But relationships with others, accomplished through communication, require that we recognise both strengths and needs. Unless we respond to a person's traits (impaired or other) as they actually **are**, rather than reacting to those which we **expect** them to have, valid relationships will become conspicuously scarce.

Appreciating the vulnerability of the population concerned, my emphasis was on minimally intrusive data collection during which the participants were entirely free to take part in or withdraw from social interaction with fellow residents. Staff were briefed and agreed that residents would be offered truthful explanations if they so wished.

The framework chosen for analysis is essentially ethnographic (Cotrell and Schulz 1993). In other words, speech is placed in the culture under investigation, allowing for both a socio-cultural and an interpersonal component of language without neurological phenomena being denied. Four major interdependent units of analysis (Saville-Troike 1989) will be touched on in what follows below. The "communicative setting" is here defined as an elderly people's "home" in terms of the care culture within which speaking occurs. The "speech community" is represented by a sample of 14 residents, nine of whom are quoted below. "Speech events" are loosely defined as episodes of conversation among the members of the speech community. Finally, emotive aspects of speech events are seen as key features setting the conversational tone for meaningful interaction. In addition to and beyond the literal meaning of spoken words they are often crucial to correct interpretation.

Residents in a care-full culture

The "communicative setting" investigated gave the impression, confirmed by a thorough DCM study, of a bright and homely environment, where great value was placed on creating a lively and stimulating atmosphere. On an interpersonal level, residents received a great deal of affectionate attention; distress was acknowledged and skilfully responded to; physical care frequently resulted in a social event for those involved; information relevant for the clients was being communicated courteously during the direct care process. Residents' views and tastes were invited and considered; their privacy was respected; breaches of etiquette were, at times, simply tolerated. A waving hand received a waving response, thereby turning a gesture into an act of communication. The presence of a Persian cat, invisible to most yet clearly part of one resident's reality, was acknowledged by staff making it part of a shared reality. Staff were aware that a variety of meanings could often be assigned to seemingly "incomprehensible" behaviour.

These are all strong indicators that the care culture is person-centred (Kitwood 1993) and that the impact of the quality of relationships (Coupland et al 1991) is recognised – relationships, that is, between carers and residents as well as between the residents themselves. When recognition failed, residents were introduced to each other. They were seen to be walking together, holding hands, assisting each other, eg getting up from a chair, moving away from obstacles. Opportunities for relationship formation among residents were clearly present, and their importance appreciated.

Out of the 10 residents mapped during the final and major DCM evaluation, seven were involved as participants throughout the period of recording and observation for this study. In total, nine women and five men, aged between 59 and 90, participated in the study; the figures were representative of those for the total nursing home population. The length of the participants' stay in the newly built home varied between several weeks and several years.

The diagnoses were carried out according to DSM-III-R criteria, and include persons probably suffering from Dementia Alzheimer's Type (DAT), Multi-Infarct Dementia (MID), Early Onset Dementia, and, in one case, dementia of unknown aetiology combined with acute confusional states. Two participants have poor hearing; one has poor eyesight. The care planning documentations, including scores obtained from assessments using the Mini-Mental State Examination (MMSE) as well as the Norton Scale, attest to varying degrees of memory impairment and disorientation together with possibly complicating factors relating to general health.

The participants were partly selected on the basis of their ability to speak audibly, and partly according to their willingness to participate. In all cases, their native language is English. Their professional careers before retirement included landscape gardener, payroll manager, cook, actress, journalist, and a nun. Variables such as marital status, family ties and friendship relationships are similarly diverse.

On the other hand, a nursing home brings people of at least similar ages to live in close proximity. This contributes to a more homogeneous environment, which is very likely to facilitate interactions within a "speech community" whose members are otherwise rather diverse (Coupland et al 1991).

Giving the benefit of the doubt

The core data illustrating peer interaction among elderly people with dementia in face-to-face interpersonal contexts consist of 17 audio-recorded units of sometimes greatly varying duration (from approximately five to 45 minutes). Poor quality

The latest available MMSE and Norton Scale scores (regarding the mental condition) of the residents are as follows:
Barbara 22/30 (1993), B4 "alert"
Deirdre 14/30 (1992), B2 "confused"
Daphne 14/30 (1992), B2 "confused"
Deborah 6/30 (1992), B3 "apathetic"
Laura 22/30 (1993), B4 "alert"
Stanley 8/27 (1993), B4 "alert"
Graham 6/30 (1992), B3 "apathetic"
Maud 12/30 (1993), B3 "apathetic"
Hilda 12/30 (1993), B3 "apathetic".

recordings or interactions not discernible to the degree necessary for evaluation were discarded. Collected in communal areas such as the dining room, a visitors' room, the reception area, and the day room, the recordings were made at varying times throughout the day, from before breakfast to just after supper time. Some meetings occurred regularly, eg at mealtimes in the dining room; others "happened" spontaneously with two, three, or more residents approaching from different directions and sharing a moment of togetherness.

The talk that was recorded and transcribed (1) showed a great deal of determination to communicate and to retain conversational initiative, as is illustrated in the following example. During a lunchtime recording in the dining room, Barbara is sitting at the table next to Deirdre who is, overall, more dependent than her. Barbara offers to pour some more tea for Deirdre, whose hearing and vision is at times rather poor. Deirdre, however, responds by shouting for attention:

Barbara: you want some more?
? (( ))
Barbara: you want some more?
Deirdre: HELLO [shouts]
Barbara: do you want some more?
Deirdre: HELLO [shouts] - can I talk to you?

Admittedly, Deirdre violates the rules of conversational etiquette: an offer is normally accepted or (politely) refused; failing to respond will have social consequences – Deirdre is promptly reprimanded for her "neglect":

Barbara: yes, talk - don't shout; I say, would you like some more TEA - and you don't answer me
Deirdre: can I go out of here?
Barbara: you will, in time - you are having a meal now
Deirdre: [relaxes]
Barbara: [pours tea]

On the other hand, it takes a great deal of social confidence to initiate contact repeatedly. After all, not being "heard" is stressful and may lead to a loss of face. Eventually, Deirdre can express her concern and Barbara's response to her question has an obviously calming effect. In the end, Barbara completes the little tea ceremony.

Context cannot be treated as an unchanging phenomenon; in every real conversation each person's contribution modifies the context in which a subsequent contribution is understood (Lesser and Milroy 1993). Faced with an incomplete picture, we may end up defining a person as forgetful or aimlessly wandering, their behaviour as wrong or inadequate even where there is evidence to the contrary. Unless, that is, we are prepared to give the benefit of the doubt even in cases of great uncertainty, assuming resourcefulness and creativity right from the start. This next example was recorded during a very pleasant supper in a relaxed and friendly atmosphere. Staff were being kind and supportive, and none of the residents – including Daphne, Barbara, and Deborah – showed any obvious signs of distress:

Daphne: I don't know, WHERE I am -
Barbara: (( )) you like a cup of tea?
Daphne: I'd LOVE a cup of tea
Barbara: yeah? I give you one - in a minute, when I get a cup
Daphne: WHERE can I get a cup?
Barbara: WAIT a minute, I'll get you one.

Barbara gets up and leaves the table, making a few steps in one direction, pausing, looking around, turning to the side and proceeding in a slightly different direction. At that point, a member of staff who is assisting a resident a few tables away, notices Barbara walking in the dining room:

Nurse: Barbara?
Barbara: yes?
Nurse: will you sit down, please?

The nurse's tone of voice is friendly but firm, and the utterance has the desired effect: Barbara returns to her seat. Up until then, Deborah had been following the events alert and with interest yet without making any comments. When Barbara sits down again, Deborah turns towards her and addresses her smilingly:

Deborah: you are a good girl [affectionate tone of voice]
Barbara: (( ))
Deborah: yes [soft voice]
Barbara: ((you come))? they won't let me give you a cup of tea -

This little incident may at first sight seem rather trivial. All we see is a person who is willing and able to help another person; perhaps to slip out of the role of "resident" into that of "carer"; to take on responsibility; and the offer is accepted. But before the interaction can be successfully completed, it is subverted – unwittingly and surely without malicious intent – subverted by a well-meaning intervention from a member of staff.

The possible implications may be far less trivial: in the long run, it may mean for the resident a loss of confidence. At the same time, a feeling of disempowerment, of being positioned as helpless, confused and incompetent may trigger off a de-skilling process. Normal behaviour interpreted in terms of the

---

1. <u>Transcript conventions</u>:

(( ))	not clearly intelligible speech;
[ ]	verbal and non-verbal features/comments;
CAPS	strongly stressed syllables;
-	short pauses;
= =	an utterance latching on to the previous one;
_ _	overlapping or simultaneous speech.

"disease" may eventually result in a self-fulfilling prophecy. Unless the responsibility for apparent conversational breakdowns is assumed jointly within a given culture, its less fortunate members will have to suffer the communicative consequences. In contrast, every bit of competence that is heard (or seen) now, will help to motivate the search for meaning and alternative interpretations in the future.

Awareness and feeling

Where memory is in decline, life can be lived in the present. Being confronted with the contradictions and uncertainties under which we live here and now implies an intensity which may be as painful as it can be gratifying. People with dementia retain an essential awareness – regardless of whether or not they can put it into words. Without the experience of temporal continuity, a feeling of abandonment and isolation may result (Cotrell and Schulz 1993). In the following example, Laura, Stanley, and Graham are enjoying their afternoon tea and some fruit in the visitors' room. Laura reflects on herself and her own situation in terms of change and uncertainty, her tone of voice sounding slightly melancholic:

Laura: you see me in one place one time, and another place (( )) another time
Stanley: hm
Laura: anywhere it says hello _ (( ))
Stanley: _ (( )) goes, that's how it GOES
Laura: eh?
Stanley: how it goes, isn't it? -

After a brief pause, Laura resumes the conversation, this time expanding on herself in relation to others, and their environment. When she recalls a part of her personal past and considers it in relation to her present life, a sense of loss becomes apparent. At the same time, she can appreciate the positive aspects of their situation:

Laura: never mind, we couldn't be in a nicer place, with nicer people around you
Graham: yes, exactly
Laura: we are not a too bad lot, are we [smiles] (( )) it puts a stop to everything you - er - sort of - interested in, that's all - I used to walk for miles
Graham: ah yes [soft voice]
Laura: never mind - (( )) you know - yes, nice people to look after us - I don't remember coming here, that's all - (( )) yes, home one minute, and somewhere else the next - [muses]

Graham and Stanley give only minimal responses, yet they clearly and appropriately signal their attention, and Graham in particular acknowledges Laura's frame of mind sympathetically.

A person's preferred style of emotional response

remains largely intact during dementia, even though defences may be lowered. Knowing someone's personality may help to resolve what could otherwise turn into some kind of miscommunication. The message a speaker intends to convey may not necessarily come out in logically sound terms.

This is complicated further by the fact that most words have several meanings, many sentences are ambiguous, and speech acts often serve more than one purpose. Even the most elegant transcription will leave a conversational episode to some degree fragmented. The utterance may be intelligible yet will remain partly uninterpretable in isolation. Features like tone of voice, or pattern of intonation assist in the discovery of "reasonable" behaviour by revealing, for instance, a person's mood and/or attitude. The next example features Deborah and Maud sitting and talking together in the dayroom before lunch:

Deborah: you're _ so good
Maud: _ you don't know what you're talking about
Deborah: (( )) did you - you're a good girl
Maud: ah - what d'you wanna borrow, eh? what d'you wanna borrow? - no way -

From the above transcript, it is not immediately obvious, whether Maud and Deborah are prey to a misunderstanding, or whether a compliment is received with hostility. Then again, some sort of humorous event could be in the make. But if you can see and hear that Deborah's voice sounds almost "meek", that she smiles when she looks at Maud, that Maud tries to keep a straight face while Deborah is slowly extending her hand toward Maud, you can see it is a playful joke – confirmed by the shared laughter that follows.

A fellow-resident may be able to share an experience to the same extent as an empathic carer. In the intimacy of nursing home friendships, feelings can be exchanged, views expounded and received with a sensitivity to the emotional needs of others.

The interaction in the following example takes place in the reception area, where Maud and Hilda have met by chance a few minutes before. It is triggered by Maud's noticing a scar on Hilda's leg. Maud's tone of voice shows concern and caring throughout the dialogue, and Hilda's story gradually unfolds:

Maud: you got anything, that's ((be)) hurting down there?
Hilda: _ yeah
Maud: _ I bet you have
Hilda: I KNOCKED myself, you know _ and
Maud: _ er - did you hurt?
Hilda: _ yeah (( )) there one there
Maud: _ (( )) oh, is it - is it =
Hilda: = and - ah - (( )) pram =

Maud: = (( )) - what, from somebody else's pram?
    oo_oh
Hilda: _ waiting - waiting to cross the road and another - form of _crossing (( ))
Maud: _ you DIDN'T go on your OWN?
Hilda: yeah, I DID
Maud: ooo_oh   _ oooh
Hilda: _ but my friend tells me - she was _ coming - THIS way, and I am going - THAT - way
        _ no - and she, she
Maud: _ THAT way - aah
Hilda: BUMPED into me and -
Maud: oh poor thing =
Hilda: = that's what happened

Despite Hilda's unspecific references, e.g. "there", "this way", "that way", Maud does not have the slightest trouble in following the account. Indeed, she does not need to be told the exactly specified location of the scar on Hilda's leg, as she can see it in front of her. Nor is it necessary to know precisely in which street Hilda had been walking, or in which direction, before she collided with "somebody else's pram".

Maud: ah, is it - does it still hurt?
Hilda: no - _ noo
Maud: _ oh er - oh THAT'S alright, cos if it's not THAT, you know, if it doesn't hurt, then -
Hilda: no, it's getting better
Maud: yeah, that's great =
Hilda: = it's not so painful as it was
Maud: yes -
Hilda: of course these things do happen, don't they? =
Maud: = they do, they do -

Maud's "affective sensitivity" contributes to mutual understanding which is mirrored in a supportive, well-attuned conversation right until the end.

A range of emotions displayed

It is, however, not necessarily "sweet-talk" that occurs; distress is heard, and so is frustration. Meals frequently tend to be emotionally and socially charged experiences. The ability to express a range of emotions is a matter of competence. Where judgement is held to be severely impaired, it is important to note that emotion displays (Harre 1993) are embodied evaluative judgements on what has affected the person. A display of joy expresses the judgement that whatever is the occasion for the display is valued by the joyful person. In the following example Maud, Laura, and Deborah share a dinner table. When Deborah notices staff rushing past and serving food to other residents, she addresses Laura with a relevant comment:

Deborah: one of the girls - says - they - they call (( )) - too much for them to do for - for them =

Laura: = eat your sandwich - don't you want them? -
Deborah: (( )) - which? - I don't know [yawns] - what, dear? - ((   ))
Laura: hm? [chewing food]
Maud: leave her, she wants to eat
Deborah: what?
Maud: she wants to eat, leave her - [reproachful]

Laura and Maud, having started eating their meal, do not approve of Deborah disturbing them. Yet Deborah would like to chat and fails to accept Laura's assistance and to comply with her repeated demands and detailed instructions to perform correctly. The others, in turn, ignore her invitations to join a conversation which is so obviously irrelevant to "proper" dining. "Proper" social eating, however, crucially involves communication and not merely of a task-oriented type.

Deborah: is it hot in here? - are you (( ))? - she sometimes - she (( )) with people anything -
Laura: eat your sandwich, look - (( )) - eat one of these sandwiches, look -
Deborah: oh this - [astonished]
Laura: well, they're ALL sandwiches [perplexed] (( )), you mean, isn't any of them, that you want? look, there's another one, there's another one, and there's another one -
Laura: you'll get a cup of tea, and then you ((   )) - d'you want - well - ((   ))
Deborah: what does he - what does he - say, dear? [friendly] -

When Laura's critical efforts show no result, her protest is expressed by anger; her helplessness by frustration; her tone of voice matches her facial expressions. Maud shows her contempt by talking down to Deborah as if she was addressing a naughty child. Half encouraging her ("you can do more ..."), half accusing her of deliberate misbehaviour ("... than you say you do"), Laura, too, infantilises Deborah who is thus found guilty of "spoiling everybody's meal":

Laura: eat your sandwich, dear [impatient], or do you want - I don't know WHAT you DO want [frustrated]
Deborah: I don't know, dear [kind]
Laura: well - eat THOSE then [angry] - look, like I am - look, there's your hand - put it in your hand
Deborah: which hand? [calm]
Maud: oh - _ don't be silly - don't be silly [contemptuous]
Laura: _ any - any hand - look, eat your san- - like we - one - two - three - (( )) look - you can do more than you say you do, you know - you spoil everybody's meal [angry] - (( )) have a sandwich, like I am

Relatively unconcerned about the tension that her behaviour apparently causes, Deborah makes her contributions to the interaction, both verbally and by (non-)action. Though not fulfilling obligations of propriety as expected by her companions, she nevertheless could be seen as helping to maintain the flow of interaction. Besides, by responding calmly and in kindness, she certainly respects conventions of politeness.

Deborah: ah yeah [friendly, tone of voice suggests interest]
Laura: look -
Deborah: I want to be with (( )) other -
Laura: look, eat your su- - eat your tea - your supper - whatever it is [frustrated] - would you like a cup of tea in a minute?
Deborah: yeah
Laura: now, I'm not gonna say any more - I'm gonna eat my supper [patronizing]
Deborah: ((where'd)) I - out there, with people I ((know)) -
Laura: eat them - look, everybody else does - eat - eat - [chewing food] (( )) - EAT some of your sandwiches - look - there's one, there's another, there's another, and there's another - - now EAT one, like everybody else did - and - that's all I've got to say -

Finally, it is worth noting that Deborah is as sociable as she is individualistic, and habitually slow eating. In this instance, as on numerous previous occasions, she starts eating when the others are nearly finished – without help. She could thus be considered as having indirectly asserted her personal style (of eating), thereby affirming once again her integrity (Coupland et al 1991).

Anybody home?

The wide range of communicative actions and interactions to which participants contributed from their (frequently ignored) perspectives (Cotrell and Schulz 1993) and with varying degrees of involvement, attest to an enormous variety in the abilities that are sustained. Mocking, praising, swearing, reassuring, objecting, complimenting, blaming and apologising are to name but a few of those encountered.

With every utterance proposing a here-and-now definition (Coupland *et al* 1991) of the situation to which subsequent talk will be oriented, some analysis, understanding, or appreciation of a turn is invariably displayed in the next speaker's response (Coupland *et al*, 1991). The content of any conversation, however, belongs to all participants and understanding is collaboratively achieved (Lesser and Milroy 1993).

Emotions seen as a collaboration of mind and body are feeling states that allow us to exist in a state of well-being or ill-being (Mills and Coleman 1994). Where cognitive memory fails, affective memory is frequently accessible. As little as a conventional greeting followed by "how-are-yous", coloured perhaps with warmth and affection, will clearly mark a person's orientation toward others – indicating a potential for small talk, or

perhaps not so small after all. Communication is a process of relating which involves moments of discord as well as harmony. It takes as much creativity as it takes insight to deal with both if we wish to engage in ongoing relationships – cognition alone will not suffice. Interactions are what they are, but the way we interpret them may make all the difference. Where appropriate speech is considered a matter of coherence (Coupland et al 1991) the expression (and recognition) of underlying emotions can complement if not compensate for an insecure linguistic basis. A consistent display of emotional cues can thus provide the missing link within actions and interactions and a key to mutual understanding.

And if you ask how I regret that parting:
It is like the flowers falling at Spring's end
Confused, whirled in a tangle.
What is the use of talking, and there is no end of Talking,
There is no end of things in the heart.

Ezra Pound

If the new culture is about coming home, the casual enquirer might ask: "Anybody home?" This research might suggest that there is much more than meets the ear – if we are prepared to listen twice.

References:
Bohling HR (1991) Communicating with Alzheimer's Patients: an Analysis of Caregiver Listening Patterns. *Int. J. of Aging and Human Development* **33(4)** 249-267.
Cotrell V & Schulz R (1993) The Perspective of the Patient with Alzheimer's Disease: a Neglected Dimension of Dementia Research. *Gerontologist* **33(2)** 205-211.
Coupland N, Coupland J, Giles H (1991) *Language, Society and the Elderly: Discourse, Identity, and Ageing.* Blackwell, Oxford.
Coupland, N, Giles, H, Wiemann, J.M. (eds) (1991) *"Miscommunication" and Problematic Talk.* Sage Publications, Newbury Park, California.
Pound E (1975) Exile's Letter. In *Selected Poems 1908-1959.* Faber and Faber, London.
Harre R (1993) Reappraising Social Psychology: Rules, Roles and Rhetoric. *Psychologist* **1** 24-28.
Kaakinen JR (1992) Living with Silence. *Gerontologist* **32(2)** 258-264.
Kitwood T (1993) Towards a Theory of Dementia Care: the Interpersonal Process. *Ageing and Society* **13(1)** 51-67.
Kitwood T, Bredin K (1992) A New Approach to the Evaluation of Dementia Care. *J. of Advances in Health and Nursing Care* **1(5)** 41-60.
Lee VK (1991) Language Changes and Alzheimer's Disease: a Literature Review. *J. of Gerontological Nursing* **17(1)** 16-20.
Lesser R, Milroy L (1993) *Linguistics and Aphasia - Psycholinguistic and Pragmatic Aspects of Intervention.* Longman, London.
Mills MA, Coleman PG (1994) Nostalgic Memories in Dementia - a Case Study. *Int. J. of Aging and Human Development* **38(3)** 203-219.
Saville-Troike M (1989) *The Ethnography of Communication.* Blackwell, Oxford.

CHAPTER SIX — Well-being, personality and residential care

SEAN BUCKLAND

This chapter begins to explore relatively uncharted territory – the inner world of the person with dementia. Its focus is the practical understanding of individuality, so that dementia care staff may feel confident in their understanding of those in their care. Specific discussion of personality illustrates the variety of persons in residential care, and suggests how the combination of personality and residential setting can have very powerful effects on individual well-being.

*T*he movement towards individual rights and choice in healthcare has largely bypassed people with dementia. Their difficulties with memory and communication often result in their rights and their individuality being ignored, or even disputed. In contrast, the new culture of dementia care seeks to promote a person-centred approach, striving to discover the uniqueness of each individual, and promote individual rights and choice.

This chapter aims to encourage awareness of, and stimulate interest in, the understanding of individuality within residential settings. Particular attention is paid to the relationships between personhood, personality and need for support. The context for this chapter is set in a piece of ongoing research taking place in residential homes, which looks at the association between physical and social settings and individuals' well-being and ill-being.

Dementia and selfhood

Neurological impairment can have profound and damaging effects on a person's abilities and hence on their sense of self. Whether that person has recently moved to a residential home or develops dementia within that home, things stop making the same sense as they did. How this happens varies for each individual, for different abilities, and at different speeds. However, the process exposes the person to a lonely experience of failure, isolation, loss of orientation and confusion. People around may behave differently, friends withdraw or get angry, and so on.

My current research involves finding out a great deal about individuals, and how they are faring in the physical and social setting in which they live. Some of this involves observing them closely over long periods of time, and in the course of this work, both their well-being and ill-being come sharply into focus. There are a number of particular vulnerabilities to which persons with dementia are regularly exposed, which we need to take into account:

Fear of failure: The person finds that simple tasks are now hard. Doing things seem to be more trouble than they are worth, especially since these are going to go wrong. It is easier to let someone else do everything.

Lack of confidence: As things go wrong more frequently, and the person loses contact with friends and those around them, they lose confidence in themselves and their value to others.

Loneliness: As recognition of faces disappears the person feels increasingly surrounded by strangers. A sense of isolation and loneliness is common.

Feelings of disorientation: As memory for places changes, the person judges each place on what it feels like. If the atmosphere does not feel like home, they want to leave, and go home.

Confusion: Things stop making sense. To the person with dementia, the facts do not tie up. There is a split between the sense the person makes of their feelings, and the explanations or information they receive (eg "It feels like Sunday, but I was told that it is Wednesday").

It might seem impossible for any carer to be able to compensate for all this, and to enable the person with dementia to have a high quality of life. Understanding what it might be like to have dementia is an important starting point in helping people to deal with their anxieties. We should care for the person so that they feel successful, confident, supported, safe and valuable.

The fragile web of well-being

One key idea behind well-being and ill-being is that we have a set of resources and needs, which are central to ourselves; they form the very core of our being. From the moment we are born, we start to build a strength of character, while the knocks in our lives set us back.

Perhaps well-being is like a spider's web, made of carefully woven strands of strength and positive experience. Each new experience, or resolving of previous damage, allows new strands to form. These are delicate and fragile at first, and firm up as we gain in confidence and sense of value. As we meet difficult life events, we try to catch the damage in the web. If our web of strength is strong enough, it will catch and contain the pain. The greater the difficulty of the event, the more chances it has to slip through, maybe even to damage the web. As more slips through, the pile below of unresolved difficulty becomes greater. This pile then acts as a dead-weight of broken experience.

Good quality care, on the other hand, will help build and reinforce strands of well-being, and will also help integrate elements of broken experience and nurture them until they become whole. Care which fails to attend to the person can only lead to the web becoming frayed and broken, while life becomes increasingly unbearable and damaging.

The signs to look for

Knowing what to look for is an important part in the fine tuning of care practice. It allows us to make the journey into the life of someone in our care. We all have a sense of how life is when we are happy or feeling good; similarly we are also aware of the drag or pain of life when we are feeling down or hurt. The ways we behave because of these feelings are the outward signs of our well-being and ill-being.

Some examples of signs of well-being are:
• **assertiveness** – the making of choices, or standing up for oneself or others;
• **warmth and affection** – giving intimate emotional support to others or responding in kind;
• **helpfulness** – the willing or spontaneous attempt to help other people;
• **creativity and expressiveness** – in such activities as dancing, singing, artwork etc (Kitwood & Bredin 1992, Kitwood 1990).

Similarly, there are some specific indicators of ill-being, for example:
• **physical discomfort or pain** – suffering from pain can be extremely disruptive to quality of life;
• **anxiety** – being tense or nervous is a common sign of feeling unsettled and unsafe;
• **sadness, grief or loneliness** – all are linked with a sense of social isolation and if they go unsupported can be very damaging to a person;
• **anger** – where the person uses or resorts to anger, the purpose of which seems to be to destroy or intimidate;
• **apathy, withdrawal or passivity** – where the person seems to be losing contact with the social world, or the will to be independent.

Different personalities, different needs

When caring for a person, attending to that person's individuality is essential. Consider, in what way is this situation individual to you and me? How am I attending

to you as the person you are? Care needs to have fine tuning, so as to promote an equal and developing relationship between two or more people.

The concept of personality is a way of considering the individuality of people, and how they act, helping us understand how they like to go about their lives, and enabling us to guess what they want. Although the categories that are used in most personality measures are crude and open to dispute, they are helpful in making some basic distinctions. As situations around us change, so does the way we choose to respond; often however, there is a similarity in our responses from one situation to another; and that is what personality scales attempt to measure.

My research uses a measure developed by Costa and McCrae (1985), the NEO Five Factor Inventory. The scale comprises five dimensions which function to develop a picture of the differing types of personality. The dimensions are neuroticism, extraversion, openness to experience, agreeableness and conscientiousness. In very general terms, each of the dimensions may be defined as follows:

Neuroticism is the predisposition to experience negative emotions.

Extraversion is the extent to which a person is outward going, sociable and excitement seeking.

The **openness** scale measures openness to experience, both intellectual and creative, and both inner and outer worlds.

Agreeableness represents the person's orientation towards others, from egocentric and antagonistic to altruistic and helpful.

Conscientiousness is the extent to which a person is organised, self-disciplined and strong-willed. A full range is possible, from the lowest end where there is an absence of the relevant characteristics (and sometimes their opposites present instead), to strong evidence of these characteristics.

In my research, which explores the interplay between personality, personhood and care, statistical analyses are indicating five main clusters, each of which is describable in terms of certain combinations of personality. Each cluster was formed by finding people of similar profile across the five dimensions. Thus far eighty-three persons are included in this study (see Table 1 on p32).

The first cluster includes those with the lowest overall levels of well-being. This cluster is best characterised by its members showing high anxiety, and low levels of extraversion, being self-centred and difficult to relate to. Some members of the cluster show less anxiety, but show a great deal of apathy to those around them and are resistant to stimulation.

The next cluster are people who like to be alone. They like to do things their way, and the world around seems to hold only little interest. For this and the next cluster there is a great risk of being ignored. Within this cluster, those who are extremely uncomfortable in their environment show very high levels of anxiety.

The third cluster consists of average people. They have no particular aspect of personality that is outstanding, being very much in the centre of each dimension. In the home they may neither demand attention greatly, nor be sufficiently outward going to generate interest around themselves.

Cluster four includes people who are very active and work hard. They are the sort of people who are frequently on the go. There are two main types of activity, depending on the person's levels of neuroticism and extraversion. Those who are more introvert are often busy doing housework or labouring. Those who are both extravert and highly anxious may frequently seek attention from those around them. Their high levels of neediness are often a source of frustration for other residents and staff alike, and such people are often very demanding. People in both sub-clusters are seen as difficult to get on with.

Members of the fifth cluster show the highest levels of well-being. Members of the cluster are outward-going and easy to get on with. They may enjoy new experiences and are open to those around them.

It may seem that the fifth cluster represents an ideal. However, it is as important that those who prefer a more solitary, or more stable lifestyle should receive equal support and reinforcement of their well-being. This can be harder where the well-being is less obvious, and more effort is required to engage the person. It is possible, however, through creating a varied and stimulating environment, where there are choices of what to do and of the extent of personal involvement.

Considering the variety of personality in this kind of way can be useful in helping tailor a setting to accommodate the needs of different types of person. Of particular importance is the interplay between a person and the situation they are in. Each individual brings their unique personality, and responds to their current situation as they understand it. This means that the way a person is acting will always be in part due to the atmosphere and situation (in the residential home or other setting).

Bearing these two aspects in mind helps us to understand a person's specific actions. Consider, for example, how we communicate, and the implication of this for dementia sufferers.

How we communicate

In day to day living, the world around us affects us, and we have an effect back. We receive signals from around us. These can be physical, social, psychological, emotional, or spiritual. We interpret these signals, often without being aware of doing so, and always in our way, influenced by all our life to date. This combination of experience and interpretation allows us to act. As neurological damage or some similar illness affects us we lose strength in our actions and we lose our capacity for understanding. This is confusing and we lose confidence in the actions we do make.

The challenge for those who care for a number of people with failing mental powers is that a personalised and fluid response is necessary for every individual. This can be hard work and requires great resourcefulness and creativity. Each person makes sense of each moment, in some way, differently. Careful attention to another's actions can guide our understanding of how they make sense of the world around them. For many of us, however, our main experience is of seeing our point of view. The move from imposing our views to successfully gauging those of another is a difficult and necessary skill.

For people whose mental powers are failing, and who have good cause to feel anxious already, there is a high risk of their feeling insecure or unsafe, wherever they are. Living with feelings such as anxiety, fear or anger is extremely damaging to the web of well-being, and can make quality of life miserable, but it is not enough to look just for signs of well- and ill-being. Both the signs of well-being and ill-being give us information about how the person feels about their immediate situation.

For example, consider members of the second cluster, those who like to be alone. Typically they do not like too much company, or too many people around; independent and solitary activity is generally preferred, and personal space is very important. The residential home environment sets many challenges to people of this type; they face the threat imposed by communal living, regularly having their personal space

Cluster	1	2	3	4	5
Primary characteristics:	High neuroticism	Low extraversion	Average on all dimensions	Very low agreeableness	Low neuroticism
	Low extraversion	Low openness		High conscientiousness	Very high extraversion
		Risk of very high neuroticism			High agreeableness
People in each cluster	30%	12%	39%	12%	7%

Table 1. Combinations of personality characteristics (n=83).

invaded by strangers, and maybe exposure in large public spaces. If in this situation they are highly anxious, withdrawn and apathetic; this is very understandable.

The residential home needs to take account of all this. Continuing the example of people in the second cluster, they are likely to want easy access to private and personal space. They may not want to join in the activities, but may prefer to watch from nearby with no pressure to participate. It may be too anxiety-provoking to sit in large open spaces, especially if the place is noisy, and so sitting with something quiet to do, like a jigsaw or reading, is preferable.

Close relationships still play a crucial role for members of this cluster, as with any other. While exuberant sociability and excitement may not play a large role in their daily life, a sense of trust and having someone near is likely to be central; they need stable and enduring relationships, as do all human beings.

Regardless of the personality of a resident, there will always be signals when a place does not feel safe enough, or not stimulating enough, or too exposing. There may be signs of all of these, often all at once, where there are several people with dementia with different personalities. In developing a safe, stimulating and personal atmosphere we need to make sure we access the person's well-being as well as minimising their ill-being.

While research into well-being and personality are still in their infancy, using ideas such as I have outlined as a guide to care appears to work at all levels of ability and severity of dementia. It does seem that the greater the well-being for most individuals, the easier it is to get on with them. Therefore, while it is harder, it is particularly necessary to build close links with those who have lower levels of well-being. Getting to know the person is the first crucial step in creating a positive, active and healthy place in which to live. For this we need as much information as we can get hold of - this helps us interpret and understand.

Dependency and intimate care-giving

One of the more complex aspects of care-giving can be enabling a person to live independently, despite physical, emotional or mental frailties. Dementia itself has an uneasy relationship with the level of dependency a sufferer may face. While cognitive decline may reduce the amount of skills a person has, it in no way reduces their basic human needs or rights. There is no clear evidence linking level of cognitive decline with loss of ability to act. Some people with severe cognitive deficits retain certain high level skills, while others, with only minimal losses, become highly dependent on support.

Thus how the residential environment deals with dependency is clearly important in the care of people with dementia. There is a risk that residential care can reduce the opportunities a person has for living independently, and indeed this could make the situation worse, speeding up the dementing process.(Kitwood 1993). However, the residential environment provides a great and appropriate opportunity for independent living for people suffering from dementia. This is because there is a communal setting with a variety of people, including staff, all with different abilities and needs. Thus the inter-relationships within the home provide a setting where people may live together with maximum independence.

Relationships are the basis of social life, and are for many the most important aspect of living, after a basic level of physical safety is achieved. The insecurity and loneliness of a dementing illness make the interpersonal relationship the most important aspect of care, and it is necessary to understand insecurity and loneliness as personal vulnerabilities. These therefore require immediate and skilled care, as much as needing help in dressing, bathing, eating or going to the toilet.

The carer, in helping, needs to accept the responsibility of being intimate with that person, for all these situations necessitate great closeness. There is a difficulty for the carer, because in each situation the nature and boundaries of that intimacy must be set by the dependent person. The carer continually needs to develop their relationship with each person they help, so that the person gains the sense that they are receiving intimate support from a trusted friend, and feels less frail, vulnerable, alone and exposed.

Developing mindfulness in care work

Person-centred care is not mechanical. We cannot diagnose a particular problem of dementia, and thus prescribe a certain action to treat the problem. It is more of an art, requiring imagination and creativity. Each person brings their own style, related to their particular personality, and this is an essential part of the dementia care process. The aim is to develop a wide variety of skills. Ultimately we seek to fit what we have to offer to the personality and needs of the resident so closely that the relationship is truly unique. When there is someone for whom we have little to offer, we can still create a respectful relationship.

Sometimes it is possible to build up a view of a person with dementia that seems to fit the facts, only to discover later that our understanding was incomplete. Those giving care need to be flexible about their ideas, and be able to view each situation from a number of perspectives. Regularly reviewing and discussing thoughts helps keep them fresh and up to date.

Ellen Langer's concept of **mindfulness** (1989) is central to giving person-centred care. She holds that mindfulness is a process of flexibility, openness and attentiveness to ideas and experience. This approach allows us to change our expectations, and makes it possible to go far beyond what we think of as our limits. In contrast mind*less*ness is restrictive of such care – that is we come to depend on standard ways of thinking developed in patterns of experience, and hold on to them when they are out of date.

While interacting with others, relationships will form naturally. Some of these relationships will be good and some poor. By being mindful, we have some potential to guide the formation of our relationships. So, ideally, in care we develop all our relationships to be personal and nourishing, and some may indeed be therapeutic. Mindfulness can be summarised in terms of four verbs: *Think, feel, understand, do.*

Think	– about what we know about each person
	– about what they are expressing.
Feel	– how we are feeling
	– how it feels to be together.
Understand	– how they might be feeling.
Do	– respond to the person
	– enable them to make choices
	– support them in feeling valuable
	– encourage their "action", on their terms
	– treat them as a (close) friend
	– help them feel at home/on holiday, etc.

Personality and the new culture

In this chapter I have mainly been discussing the role of personality in the caring relationship. I have set out a need for the development of specific relationships between carer and person with dementia that take into account each individua's personhood, the variety of personality and the abilities of the carer. These ideas about personality and personhood have been developed in recognising that people express themselves through specific and identifiable behaviours, and that these behaviours will be in part due to their current situation.

Preliminary research findings are suggesting that there may be five broad clusters that describe the range of personality types presently observable in today's residential care settings. This approach is useful both in the understanding of the social situation in the home, and in identifying unhelpful aspects of the residential culture. The role of care staff is described as including a responsibility for developing fine-tuned and sensitive relationships; and the role of the residential home is to create space for each person to have a way of life that is authentically their own.

While there is a growing interest in person-centred care and concern for the psychological well-being of residents with dementia, there is still a large shortfall in the awareness and the complex skills this involves. When personality and social situation have properly been taken into account, we will be much closer to having developed the New Culture of Care.

References

Costa PT, McCrae RR (1985) *The NEO Personality Inventory.* Psychological Assessment Resources Inc, Odessa, Florida.

Kitwood T (1993) Person and Process in Dementia. *International Journal of Geriatric Psychiatry* **8** 541-545.

Kitwood T (1990) The Dialectics of Dementia: With Particular Reference to Alzheimer's Disease. *Ageing and Society* **10** 177-196.

Kitwood T, Bredin, K (1992) Towards a Theory of Dementia Care: Personhood and Well-Being. *Ageing and Society* **12** 269-287.

Langer, EJ (1989) Minding Matters: The Consequences of Mindlessness-Mindfulness. *Advances in Experimental Social Psychology* **22** 137-173.

CHAPTER SEVEN | Sexuality and sexual needs of the person with dementia

CAROLE ARCHIBALD

Sexuality and dementia can be difficult for staff to contemplate. It is often seen as a problem area. Using the framework for action suggested here, a more positive approach can be taken – one that addresses the needs of all concerned including the person with dementia. This problem-solving strategy offers staff a structure to work with, at the same time guiding them towards a more person-centred approach. It also asks staff to look at their own experience and attitudes.

Sexuality and dementia – whatever next? The idea of associating the two issues seems bizarre to many people; a source of amusement. Generally there has been a failure to consider the sexual needs of people with dementia, and by extension, those of carers. The fact that people with dementia might have sexual needs and form relationships, is a relatively recent idea which can be difficult to contemplate.

Tony Gibson (1992) comments "Old people are generally regarded as 'past it' and consequently not of fully adult status, to be pitied and patronised." This view has extended to people with dementia and has brought out a huge sense of parenting and responsibility in us. They have been considered as somehow different. For some people it involves a great leap of attitude to consider people with dementia as sexual beings – beings similar to the rest of us. On admission to long term care their identity, including their sexual identity, has often been shed and left at the front door.

Slowly but surely, ideas and attitudes are shifting. Pre-eminent in the new culture of care is an acknowledgement of the uniqueness of each person with dementia and the acceptance that they are similar beings to ourselves. Here problem behaviours are seen as attempts to communicate need.

The new culture demands that we explore the personhood of the person with dementia. Ideally before we do that we need to acknowledge our own sense of personhood; to value and care for ourselves and understand our own psychological make-up. Nowhere is this more true than in the area of sexuality.

What is sexuality?

But firstly, what is meant by sexuality? Sexuality is part and parcel of our being; we are in fact sexual in every way, all the time. Sexuality is part of what makes each of us unique and special (Stuart & Sundeen 1979). It is an interlinking aspect of our lives rather than a discrete and separate entity. Sexuality is about being human. It embraces such things as close relationships, physical and psychological closeness, kissing and hugging as well as sexual intercourse. For many people it is reflected in how we present ourselves to the world, our self esteem, our self confidence, what we wear; and how we look.

Never before has sexuality, in a limited and narrow sense, been so overtly portrayed in our society. While we have never been so assailed with media images of sexuality in books, in the cinema and in our daily papers, these images are primarily of young people. Older people are virtually invisible when it comes to the portrayal of sexuality. Paradoxically, while the whole subject of sexuality is publicly proclaimed it nevertheless remains for us as individuals, whether young or old, a private concern. We do not tend to talk about our own sexuality, and our own sex lives. We seldom explore our attitudes and prejudices and look at where they originate.

Our own attitudes

We have all inevitably been influenced by the society and the culture in which we live. Our views are often related to how and what we were told about sexuality by our parents. Unwittingly we have absorbed many attitudes towards sexuality from them and those people of significance around us during our most impressionable and formative years.

How the expression of sexuality was portrayed matters in a number of ways – primarily because it will tend to reflect how we address the expression of sexuality by those we care for. It is not hard to imagine that where it was seen as a shameful thing, attitudes are going to be less than positive.

If we believe in a holistic approach and in the new culture of care, in caring for people with dementia, then expressing sexuality is a component of that care. Most assessment forms, whether nursing or social work, include a section on the expression of sexuality, yet how many people fill in that aspect of the care plan? How many feel comfortable including sexuality? How many people discuss it with both people with dementia and/or their carers?

Often the expression of sexuality by people with

dementia in long term care is seen as problematic, seldom as a positive aspect of a person's life. The subject is fraught and complex. It often causes great consternation and concern in staff. What many staff have asked for is some kind of guide to help them through this difficult and precarious area. They need a frame of reference to help them start talking about and addressing the issue of sexuality and sexual needs.

Problem-solving approach

If sexuality is seen as problematic there might be some advantage in approaching the whole area from that perspective. A problem solving approach which allows issues to be examined, one which taps into, and uses staff's expertise, would be useful. The framework for action opposite, discussed in my book *Sexuality and Dementia: A Guide* (Archibald 1994) offers such an approach. It is essentially a stop, look and listen approach. The framework allows a careful analysis of issues using a structured approach.

Some might ask, how is this compatible with the new culture of care? It is compatible in that the "problem" is not seen as belonging simply to the person with dementia, rather it explores who is the problem for: the staff; the carer; other residents; the person with dementia or the organisation? It asks, is there indeed a problem? It will assist in working out a plan of action so that the needs of all the people involved can best be met.

The framework for action will be used in the case study example below, to tease out some of the difficulties and possible courses of actions to take. Most people will identify with some or all of the aspects in this case study.

Mr A, a man in his 70s, was admitted to residential care as his wife was finding it increasingly difficult to manage him at home. She visits him twice a week at the residential home. When she visits she is constantly finding fault with members of staff. The staff consequently have started to avoid her where possible. Mr A is proving difficult too for the staff. He is behaving in a sexually explicit way. The staff have made complaints to the manager and asked that Mr A be given something to sedate him.

Analysing the behaviour

Description of the behaviour. Firstly there is a need to say simply what the behaviour is so that everyone is able to understand what the issues are.

So the description might read: "Mr A is always trying to put his hands up the skirts of staff's dresses and grabbing their breasts when they are attending to his toileting needs. He also puts his hands up the skirts of other residents."

In a situation like this it can be useful to establish frequency of these unsolicited actions and to find out if there is any pattern to what is happening. Some people argue that it is a lot of trouble to note down every time the behaviour occurs, especially when there are few staff on duty. This needs to be acknowledged so that some negotiation can take place as to what is realistic. It might be that the information can be written down when a member of staff is giving out medicines, and at handover times. Whatever is decided on, it will soon become clear that the exercise is worthwhile in giving insight into the pattern. It helps to prevent the "Mr A is always doing" syndrome.

Once the **pattern** and the **frequency** have been established then it is useful for staff to look at what were the **triggers**, the reasons for the behaviour taking place. What was happening in the room at the time, what behaviour resulted and what where the consequences.

Is there a problem?

Once the behaviour has been thoroughly described, the next question to be asked is: "Is there a problem?" If there is not, no further action need take place. If yes there is a need to establish who finds it a problem.

For whom is it a problem?

Is it a problem for the organisation? It might be that the reputation of the organisation is compromised, that carers complain about their relatives being sexually harassed. It might be that staff are complaining of harassment. Is sexuality rigidly repressed? Does the old culture of care exist where only basic needs are attended to, where the day is punctuated simply by mealtimes and toilet rounds? Are there too few activities? Are people including Mr A, utterly bored with the daily routine?

What about staff? Is it a problem for them; a problem for all staff? Are younger staff targeted? Do staff see this harassment as part and parcel of their job or the opposite? Is it something they feel they should not have to put up with? Is there a need to set limits and protect staff while at the same time understanding the reasons for the behaviour; the needs being expressed by Mr A?

Are staff by their actions contributing to the situation, by using humour inappropriately, leaning over Mr A in an unbefitting way? Sometimes we treat people with dementia as asexual beings, as children, and perhaps lean over or behave in ways we would not do with younger men. If staff have perceived Mr A in this light, then there can be great consternation when he starts to act as a sexual adult.

Are staff, as a result of this man's actions, avoiding him where possible and giving the minimum amount of touch and attention?

Asking these questions allows staff attitudes and reactions to be explored and is an opportunity for staff to give vent to their feelings, so that some constructive work can take place.

Is it a problem for family carers?
Little is known about how family carers cope, particularly partners or spouses. The subject of sexuality is seldom discussed. The nature of a couple's relationship before the onset of dementia, and the differences dementia has made to the relationship, may need to be explored further.

Mr A's wife seldom if ever touches him when she visits. She also seems to find difficulty in accepting the diagnosis of dementia. For many carers there is loss and grief to be worked through. Carers are often reluctant to discuss any difficulties, for example feelings of revulsion, excessive sexual demands or the role reversal aspect of the relationship. If staff are uncomfortable too when discussing sexuality, an *impasse* can develop.

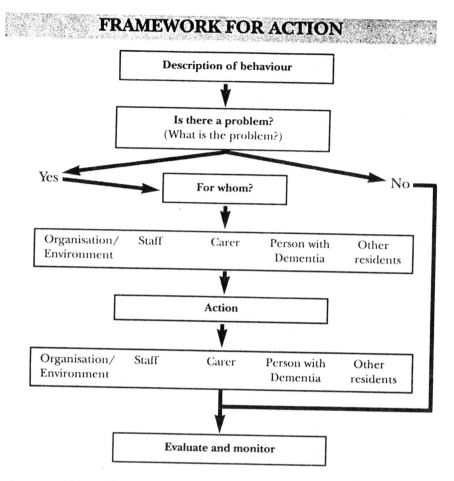

FRAMEWORK FOR ACTION

Description of behaviour

Is there a problem?
(What is the problem?)

Yes — For whom? — No

Organisation/Environment — Staff — Carer — Person with Dementia — Other residents

Action

Organisation/Environment — Staff — Carer — Person with Dementia — Other residents

Evaluate and monitor

Other residents also enter the equation. Many people with dementia are cared for in non specialist settings. Residents are expected to tolerate an assortment of difficult situations. In Mr A's case, are other residents being intimidated and exploited? Are they distressed by his advances? Have they complained? Have they ridiculed him? Have they welcomed his advances?

Lastly **the person with dementia:** how does he or she fare in this situation? Often the need for sexual expression is frowned upon. Often it is not allowed in residential care. In the new culture of care however, instead of simply seeing the problem as a manifestation of dementia, it is seen as a way of expressing need.

So what are the needs being expressed? Is Mr A getting enough attention, enough touch? In many cases people with dementia are only touched when there is a task to do, such as bathing. We all need touch in differing degrees. It is necessary for our physical as well as our emotional well-being.

Is Mr A misrecognising staff, thinking one of them is his wife? It is worthwhile for staff to pause at this juncture and try to think what his needs might be, and why he is expressing them this way.

Developing an action plan

As we are proposing a person-centred approach, with the maintenance of personhood being at the core of the action plan, then we should start with Mr A:

The person with dementia – Mr A: In the field of dementia it can be a novel idea to see the expression of sexuality as a good thing, contributing to the individual's sense of identity and sense of personal well being, as something which empowers a person, rather than a problem. Those people with a good sense of self, who have self-esteem, are powerful people. According to Anthony Giddens (1992) sexual freedom follows power and is an expression of it. If we accept this statement, we need to ask how powerful are older people, especially people with dementia in residential care?

Equally we need to ask, how appropriate is it for them to express what are normally seen as private actions, in a public place, albeit now their home? The expression of sexuality is a basic human right – that is so long as it does not infringe the rights of others. In Mr A's situation, other people's rights are seen to be infringed, so how should we best address his needs?

If his behaviour is to be interpreted as a means of expressing need, could that need be one of attention, closeness, a need for touch? If this interpretation of Mr A's actions is correct then what he has achieved is the very opposite of his intentions, of what his needs are. His wife avoids touching him, staff avoid him and other residents are taken out of his reach or also avoid him. So, are there ways of giving him legitimate touch? For those staff who feel able, what about giving him some time; time talking to him, time encouraging pride in appearance, time to give a hand massage.

If Mr A is able, dancing is good as it provides a chance for touching and being held. Going on an outing where there is a chance to dress up and feel good is useful. Having an opportunity to choose what to wear helps give a person a sense of control and gives some power back to that person. Collecting biographical information can help in discovering so much about the person, aspects which really matter. The problem needs to be re-framed and seen in the context of that person's life.

The family carer – Mrs A – seems to be experiencing difficulties in being close to her husband. Is it possible for a member of staff to explore past and present relationships with her? It can help to use such phrases as "I appreciate it may be difficult for you to talk about this" or "Some people have found that dementia has had a dramatic effect on their sexual lives."

It needs to be said that there has to be a trusting relationship built up before these issues can be explored. Also Mrs A seems to have had difficulty with her husband's diagnosis of dementia so there may be a need to explore this first, offering her an opportunity to give vent to her feelings. It may be possible after this to engage her in the care plans to help Mr A.

The issue of whether to involve carers when discussing a person's sexuality needs to be discussed. Will it help or hinder the situation? Can the spouse/partner help? As to involving the person's children, old people do not normally discuss their sex lives with their children – should it be the case now? It might seem to be crossing boundaries. What could it achieve? (Baikie 1992)

Staff: If staff are to be involved in helping the person with dementia and their carers, they need to feel comfortable with their own sexuality. Workshops and training to explore issues are a good starting point. Sexuality is a part of all our lives. It goes hand in glove with our spiritual, psychological and emotional needs. This applies to us all. Being involved in this area of work, what has become apparent is that issues can be the same for staff and the person with dementia.

One case in point is that of sexual abuse. This has impact whether in the previously locked up long-term memory of the person with dementia, or in staff who themselves have been abused. Often these issues have not been explored. They will certainly affect the way staff approach and deal with the expression of sexuality by people in their care. The expression of sexuality by people with dementia can trigger memories for staff. It goes without saying that issues like this need to be explored sensitively by those experienced in counselling.

There are many other issues for staff which this brief chapter cannot discuss, issues such as legal aspects and risk taking. How do staff stand in relation to the law if they intervene or do not intervene? Suffice to say that in the context of the law the collection of information and a detailed care plan which demonstrates that the best needs of the person are being served, is helpful.

Collecting detailed information and deciding on who are the necessary people to be involved is important. This is so that the most intimate details of the one or two people involved are not made widely available. The care plan can then be drawn up. It is also important that the measures decided on are in the person's best interests and not simply in the interest of staff. It vital that all staff adhere to the plan so that there is a consistent approach.

Other residents: In Mr A's case, the measures discussed might go some way towards improving the situation. Equally it is helpful to speak to other residents involved and acknowledge their feelings, and where possible encourage staff to give some thought to the situation. Can the other residents involved suggest ways of helping? It might be that with staff support they could set limits, perhaps telling Mr A that the behaviour is unacceptable.

The organisation: Resources are often a central issue. Sometimes there are few resources available for such things as activities, training for staff and facilities so that if a carer wished they could have a meal and stay overnight with their partner. If resources are not available, are there innovative ways of using existing facilities? By using folding beds or chair beds, partners can be accommodated overnight if that is their wish. Could creating a private area in the living area enable couples to have some privacy? Are there such things as settees in the sitting area?

Monitoring and evaluation

As in the compilation of any care plan, it is imperative that time is given to monitor and evaluate the process. Have the interventions been successful, do they need some fine tuning or is there a need to consider a radical new approach? The "problem" is unlikely to go away, so it is important that it is addressed until it has been resolved for the person with dementia and where possible the other people involved.

The essence of each person

If we are committed to the view that sexuality is a vital and integral part of our being, then we need to pay much closer attention to the way it is expressed by each individual with dementia, and we must take particular care to acknowledge each one as an adult thinking, feeling being. It is easy when caring for a large number of people with dementia to lose a sense of each person's individuality and adulthood, but if quality care is aspired to, this is what is required.

Staff need to find ways to discover the essence of each person; life story books are a good starting point.

From this can stem a sense of the person's past, their relationships past and present and thus a sense of their sexual identity. It can be likened to pieces of a large jigsaw puzzle, the pieces of which go together to make up that unique human being. If we are serious about promoting a new culture of care then facilitating the expression of a person's sexuality has to be to the fore in that care, if that is what the person wishes.

In this chapter I have explored ideas and looked at alternatives to reaching out for extra sedation or transferring a person to hospital. The ideas discussed here here do not provide an easy option. They do in fact require more work and a good honest look at ourselves; our own history and attitudes to sexuality, and the way these may affect our responses to the expression of sexuality in our workplace.

The benefits that accrue however from this strategy are worth the effort. Staff have a more structured approach which lends direction and gives a sense of support. The needs of all concerned are addressed – a new culture of care in effect.

References

Archibald C (1994) *Sexuality and Dementia: A Guide.* Dementia Services Development Centre, Stirling.

Charnock A (1994) *Sexuality and Patient Care.* Chapman and Hall, London.

Gibson T (1992) *Love, Sex and Power Place.* Freedom Press.

Stuart GW and Sundeen SJ (eds) (1979) *Principles and Practice of Psychiatric Nursing.* C.V. Mosby, St Louis. Quoted in Ooijen E, Giddens A (1992) *The Transformation of Intimacy.* Polity Press, Oxford.

Baikie L (1992) Personal communication.

CHAPTER EIGHT | Broadening our approach to spirituality

ELIZABETH BARNETT

Spirituality and dementia presents a far broader agenda than "assessing and attempting to meet the spiritual needs of persons with dementia". We cannot separate the spiritual needs of the caregiver and the cared for. Without limiting ourselves to any particular faith tradition, we may all use the resources of our own inner journey to resource our "care" with "love".

*B*oth spirituality and dementia bring us face to face with how we define ourselves as human beings. Are we no more than the sum total of our physical and cognitive functioning? And what is left when, in particular, the latter fails us? The way in which we interact (or not) with those whose intellectual powers are failing them might seem to indicate that we do not view them as quite as "human" as ourselves. At an individual level this means that we may fail to take seriously their distress, or at a societal level to provide the care and support which a genuine respect for their personhood would require of us. Yet if we accept that each and every one of us is a being with spiritual dimensions, then we can no longer justify a "them and us" attitude to persons with dementia.

"Spirituality and dementia", therefore, presents a far broader agenda than "assessing and attempting to meet the spiritual needs of persons with dementia". This is, however, rightly a focus of concern for those whose work highlights for them the inadequacy of understanding of the inner lives of many persons with dementia receiving care in residential settings. While this deficit in individual assessment obviously needs to be addressed in any care environment, it is not in itself more than a symptom of the "world view" of our culture. This world view includes neither an acceptance of the coherence of all aspects of a person – both outward and inward – nor the definition of "personhood" in terms of relationship rather than role. Yet our spirituality is about finding the "one-ness": perceiving our place in creation, our relationship to "the ground of our being" (or as some of us would say, God, the Spirit) and to each other. Thus we cannot separate the spirituality of the caregivers and the cared for. How, in any case, may we seek to address the spiritual needs of those with dementia without recognising our own?

We may begin with a definition of terms. The new culture of dementia care necessarily involves a new interpretation of "dementia", seeing it in terms of what it means to the whole person – both the person with the dementing illness and the person "caring" for him or her – rather than merely focusing on a disease process.

In defining "spirituality" we may avoid being anchored in any one faith tradition. Indeed, "received religion" can too often be misunderstood as providing ready-made answers which obviate the need for individual discovery. Yet is is only from our own personal inner journey that we can acquire that understanding which we can meaningfully share with others. Jung tells us that every inner journey is a spiritual journey, whether it is explicitly so recognised or not (Storr 1983).

Let us therefore remove from our consideration of "Spirituality" any pre-conceived concepts of "Religion" in its social, cultural and institutional manifestations. Instead we may substitute that universal personal search for meaning and coherence known to each and every one of us in our moments of distress and decision, of joy and wonder. We often refer to these as "moments of truth". These are the times of questioning the incomprehensible, wrestling with the insoluble, and of sensing that we are beckoned to reach out beyond the boundaries of self into that gentler dimension where our individuality is merged into a sense of completeness and belonging.

It is not necessary to attach formal religious labels to these experiences. But it is, perhaps, important to recognise that they form a fundamental commonality of individual human lives, and as such a potential basis for mutual understanding. In this sense we may all describe ourselves as spiritual beings, and in this way approach our subject of the relationship of spirituality to the new culture of dementia care.

A false sense of separation

In that part of my own inner journey which has run parallel to my work among those with dementia and those who care for them I have found these words of Mary's song of praise (the Magnificat) from the Christian New Testament particularly helpful: "He hath scattered the proud in the imagination of their hearts." *Luke 1:46-55.*

Who are the proud? They are those who characterise themselves, implicitly or explicitly, by their sense of superiority – of difference and separateness from others. They feel themselves superior (and therefore separate) because of what they possess that others do not, and of what they can do that others cannot. They differentiate themselves from the "abnormality" of others, the handicaps and disabilities (especially where these involve problems of communication) which challenge the ease of the "normal". Sin, in classical Christian theology, is separation from God. Pride is the sin which separates us from God and from our own "spiritual self" (Israel 1976) by separating us from other people.

Within our context of dementia care, then, we may ask ourselves whether we are "the proud" – the "normal" people who disdain persons with dementia already humbled through a degenerative neurological process. Yet implicit in our seeking to address their spiritual needs is an acceptance of them as fellow spiritual beings. How can we justify, therefore, a hierarchical psychology in our approach to care – an "us and them" perspective? and if we cannot justify it, how can we work to undermine it within ourselves?

Through loving imagination

It is here that the song of Mary provides us with an answer, for the good news is that "the proud" are not heartless. Indeed it is precisely through "the imagination of their hearts" that their pride may be scattered (to paraphrase). This wonderful expression: "the imagination of their hearts," gives us a rich synonym for compassion.

It is not through our objective perception or intellectual understanding of others that we can bridge the gap of separation to reach them. It is through our deepest feelings and our own experience of suffering that the imagination of our hearts (which can be so proud, greedy, fearful and deceitful) can be informed and transformed, so that it becomes a loving and compassionate imagination.

The power which the song of Mary praises is that power to transform each individual from within. In this way we can "suffer with" (the literal meaning of sympathy) those who may not be able to communicate their suffering to us without our having travelled our own part of the way to meet them.

To travel alongside the suffering of another, to take turns in bearing his or her burden, is also to feel his or her pain. No wonder "the proud" have a vested interest in safeguarding their separateness. In entering the world of a person with dementia we are faced with the fact that a person continues in a feeling existence despite the gradual disintegration of mind and often of

body. We would rather believe that such a person was no longer aware, in some sort of living anaesthesia.

Yet to open our hearts to that person is to open also our eyes and our minds so that we are forced to realise that this is not the case. What a strange, frustrating and often frightening place their world must be, bereft as we so often leave them of the comfort of our companionship; and for one out of every five of us who reach the age of eighty, this is how our world will be. Where can we find the courage, then, to face this reality which surrounds us in every dementia care environment? What can fuel the imagination of our hearts?

"Listen to what love requires of you" (Quaker Faith and Practice 1994)

Care has become the language of the social sciences; indeed, our subject is the new culture of dementia *care*. *Love*, however, is the language of the spirit: "Love ye one another as I have loved you" (*John 15:12*). Love is that gift of the spirit which wells up from deep within us – from "that of God"/"our higher self"/the transpersonal self, whatever the language we use to describe the wellspring of our being, our essence, our divine spark. This is the core or ground of our being which is not subject to the changing influences of the world, although the vicissitudes of life may blow the window open so that the soul may see out more clearly. Delving into our own deeper selves we may find the love we need to inform "the imagination of our hearts".

How do we do this? Our own experience of suffering may, if we let it, open doors within us through which love may flow out to those fellow sufferers with whom we can learn to share our sense of powerlessness. Henri Nouwen wrote in his book, "The Wounded Healer":

"...no one can help anyone without becoming involved, without entering with his whole person into the painful situation, without taking the risk of becoming hurt, wounded or even destroyed in the process ... (without a willingness) to make one's own painful and joyful experiences available as sources of clarification and understanding... The great illusion of leadership is to think that man can be led out of the desert by someone who has never been there" (Burnell 1989a).

This paradox of the transforming quality of suffering, then, is both our challenge and our promise, our fear and our reassurance, our port and our adventure. It is through our own vulnerability – our sensitivity to our own suffering, our brokenness and our inadequacies – that we find our "higher self", the divine spark within us, through which we can experience (not "believe" or "understand") our one-ness with others, and with God – if we choose thus to describe our spiritual life.

Learning to breathe under water

It is very difficult to explore these ideas. Everything within us cries out against facing our pain. To bring in a new metaphor, it is like walking into a great wave that is rolling towards us from the ocean, threatening to break over us and drown us. Our every inclination is to run – with the wave at our back. "The proud", then, are those who are still managing to outstrip the wave, and disdaining those behind them already engulfed. But to look backwards is to slow down: we are engulfed too if we stop to cast a compassionate glance over our shoulder, or to hold out a hand to help.

Sheila Cassidy, in her book on the spirituality of caring ("Sharing the Darkness") quotes a poem given her by a missionary sister she had known in Chile, named Carole Bialok. It is about the embracing of a seeming lack of choice in the way that suffering and pain arrive in our lives without our being able to hold them at arm's length, and also about how this can be the metaphor for another embrace – how God breaks through into our consciousness. The poet describes how she built her house ("a strong house") beside the sea. It was built firmly on rock, not on shifting sand, and the poet and the sea remained respectful neighbours – "keeping our distance" – with the sands between them:

> And then one day
> (and I still don't know how it happened)
> The sea came.
> Without warning.
> Without welcome even.
> Not sudden and swift, but a shifting across the
> sand like wine,
> less like the flow of water than the flow of blood.
> Slow, but flowing like an open wound.
> And I thought of flight, and I thought of drowning,
> and I thought of death.
> But while I thought the sea crept higher
> till it reached my door.
> And I knew that there was neither flight
> nor death nor drowning.
> That when the sea comes calling you stop
> being good neighbours,
> And you give your house for a coral castle
> And you learn to breathe under water.
> (Cassidy 1988)

Sheila Cassidy explains how while she had always seen the sea in this poem as a metaphor for the presence of God moving in on our life, a monk to whom she had shown it had interpreted it as "the gradual encroachment of the agony of the world upon one's consciousness." However, she writes, "It is only now, ten years on, that I begin to understand what he meant when he said that the great mystery is that the two are really the same" (Cassidy 1988).

Those who have a near and dear one with dementia have, indeed, stopped being friendly-from-a-distance neighbours with the spiritual sea of suffering. It has invaded every aspect of their life and, while it feels like drowning, they are needing to learn to breathe under water – gulping in their own fear and pain and helplessness, so that they may swim with their near one who is floundering in a rising tide of cognitive disruption. It is not that they have chosen to go scuba-diving. The sea has chosen them not they the sea. The loyalty of love is the choice to go beyond choosing, and in that surrender we reach deeper into ourselves. It is from these depths that we may answer the call from the depths of the Other.

A new kind of gift relationship

Learning to breathe under water is one metaphor. Another is that of mining for that which is most precious deep within ourselves. That most precious of our attributes is love, and it is love which is the gift we both receive and give when we are allowed to share God's vision of another person. We see more of and in them than they see of themselves. Because love is spirit-given it focuses on the positive, creative, miraculous qualities of the loved one – that which makes them a unique child of God – their "irreplaceability".

This divine essence of the person is what remains unchanged. It is this gift which persons with dementia most need from us: the upholding and preservation of their personhood by seeing that which is unchanged and uniquely precious in them reflected in the eyes (and the behaviour) of those who love them. This is the image of themselves which is the most important gift we have to offer them. It does not show their deficits, of which they are painfully aware, and which awareness causes them fear, insecurity, and increasing confusion.

"Care", therefore, is not enough. We need love in order to be able to give to persons with dementia what they most deeply need. No wonder dementia is so feared and marginalised in our society. No wonder that dementia care is often the "Cinderella service". For dementia challenges us not just to "do-as-you-would-be-done-by" as good citizenship requires, but to become fully ourselves as loving, spiritual beings. This transformation will only come, at the individual level, from that place deep within us which is often reached only through our own brokenness, fear and confusion. And at a societal level the new culture of dementia care will only be achieved through this profound transformation of individual caregivers.

When we speak of "entering into the spirit of things" we mean by that the letting go of a "stand-offish" manner, whereby we only observe from the sidelines, and becoming instead a participant in the midst – at the heart of things. Our route from the sidelines of "care" into the midst of "love" will run through the imagination of our hearts, as we enter more honestly into the reality of our own experience of need and pain, fear and incomprehension, to find the roots of our being, our spiritual heritage. From these depths we may find a way of answering the spiritual needs of persons with dementia – not merely in ritual and denominational terms, but in ways of relating at that level where each being preserves the uniqueness of their creation, the little candle in their own house, still intact but requiring the mirror of loving eyes to be recognisable. Entering into our own spirit we enter into others, and in this way both may deepen their experience of the greater Spirit which enfolds and permeates us all.

Travelling alongside persons with dementia can be deeply challenging for paid caregivers and heartbreaking for their nearest and dearest. Yet the paradox is that it is precisely in this, our own suffering, that "the imagination of our hearts" is activated. Then our pride is scattered, our separateness disappears, and we can give that appreciation of their unique, intact divine essence which is what love shows us in the unity of the Spirit.

Strength in weakness

Broadening our approach to the subject of spirituality beyond the conventional institutional concept of religion, allows us to frame our interpretation of the spiritual needs of persons with dementia in a way that also includes the spiritual needs of all those who "care" for them. Indeed, the two are mutually dependent. To provide the loving and imaginative support for their unique personhood so needed by someone with dementia, we who care for them need to delve deep into our own spiritual resources. Merely to tinker with "services provision" and "care delivery" will not suffice.

All of us as individuals have a need to fulfill the calling of our own inner journey in order to resource our care with love. And it is through not only our own pain but that which we share with (and because of) others, that we are enabled to do this. The stripping away of intellectual functioning takes both the person with dementia and those who accompany them beyond the usual patterns of interaction and into a deeper level of communication, where soul meets soul. We may learn to use our own weakness, confusion and fear to find a way through to a new understanding both of others and of our own spirituality. This is how Teilhard de Chardin expressed it:

"When the signs of age begin to mark my body (and still more when they touch my mind); when the ill that is to diminish me or carry me off strikes from without or is born within me; when the painful moment comes, in which I suddenly awaken to the fact that I am ill or growing old; and above all at that last moment when I feel I am losing hold of myself and am absolutely passive within the hands of the great unknown forces that have formed me; in all those dark moments, O God, grant that I may understand that it is You (provided only my faith is strong enough) who are painfully parting the fibres of my being in order to penetrate to the very marrow of my substance and bear me away within Yourself" (Burnell 1989b).

Broadening our approach to spirituality can allow us to use our own suffering and that which we share with others in such a way that our own personal inner journey is illumined and enriched. It can also empower us to understand at a far deeper level the fundamental emotional survival needs of those whose very sense of identity is being continually undermined by neurological degeneration on the one hand and the defensive insensitivity of their fellow human beings ("the proud") on the other. To accept ourselves as spiritual beings is to recognise that same dimension in all our fellow humans.

The psalmist called to his God "from the depths" (Psalm 130). The bewildered dementia patient brought into an assessment ward lashes out with his stick at the door in panic and incomprehension. The elderly man with a heart condition asks how he can bear another sleepless night caring for his confused, eternally agitated and incontinent wife. The staff nurse on an understaffed "EMI" ward where sixty per cent of the patients require total physical care despairs of being able to live up to her professional ideals of providing truly individual patient-centred care. The manager whose budget has just been reduced for the second time in a year does not know how to face his staff with the decisions he has been forced to make.

For all of us the "fibres of our being" are being parted "to the very marrow of our substance". Can we feel the one-ness? Can we use our own experience of fear and frustration, confusion and powerlessness, to open the doors of compassion in our soul? And can we find in this the courage to follow the way that love requires of us? The power whose strength is made perfect in weakness is already at work within each of us.

References
Burnell S J (1989a) *Broken for Life.* Quaker Home Service, London. p30.
Burnell S J (1989b) *Broken for Life.* Quaker Home Service, London. p44.
Cassidy S (1988) *Sharing the Darkness: the Spirituality of Caring.* Darton, Longman & Todd, London. p7-9.
Israel M (1976) *Precarious Living: The Path to Life.* Mowbray, London & Oxford. p75-81.
Quaker Faith and Practice (1994) *Advices and Queries.* Yearly Meeting of the Religious Society of Friends, London. p1-6.
Storr A (1983) *Jung: Selected Writings.* Fontana, London. p 229.

CHAPTER NINE | The genetics of Alzheimer's disease: rethinking the questions

ANDREA CAPSTICK

A great deal of scientific expertise is currently being devoted to the search for a genetic basis for Alzheimer's disease. It is argued here that such research is unlikely to produce a "miracle cure" in the foreseeable future, and that, in the relentless scientific pursuit of "AD genes", the needs and concerns of people with AD and their families are being marginalised. The new culture of dementia care will put the emphasis on informed and supportive counselling in relation to genetic issues, and will foster a heightened awareness of the limitations of genetic research.

*W*hen people hear that I am carrying out research on the social and ethical aspects of the genetics of Alzheimer's disease, I have noticed that very often the first question they ask is, "Are you a geneticist?". The second question which inevitably to follows is, "Well, is there a gene for Alzheimer's disease – is it inherited?" The answer to this question, in so far as there is one, will I hope become clear in the course of this chapter. What is immediately striking, however, is that this question is obviously felt by many people to be of central importance, yet when pressed they can rarely say why. There seems to be a general, vague belief that discovering "a gene" will lead to an overnight cure, or at least the condition will be wiped out for future generations. In fact there is little evidence to support either of these speculations.

What has been brought home to me very forcibly by hearing these two questions repeated so often, is the extent to which genetic research has been allowed to set its own agenda. It is widely believed that science is not the business of ordinary people; that it should be left to experts who have access to all kinds of definitive knowledge about things which are incomprehensible to the rest of us. If vast resources in terms of time, money and expertise are being invested in the pursuit of a genetic basis for Alzheimer's disease, this must be for a good reason and who are we to question it?

This kind of deferential attitude toward science, highlighted in Tom Kitwood's chapter in this book as a feature of the old culture of dementia care, is not a healthy one. Science affects all our lives in innumerable ways, not all of them beneficial, and it is not subject to any form of democratic control. Genetic research in particular is currently advancing in directions which may soon come to have vast implications for all of us.

In moving towards the new culture of dementia care there is a need to develop what one radical geneticist has described as "a reasonable scepticism" toward scientific research and its sometimes grandiose claims (Lewontin 1993). We need to allow genuine human concerns to set the agenda and rethink the questions we ask about genetic research into Alzheimer's disease. In the course of this chapter I have raised some of the questions I think we ought to be asking.

Is it really a single disease?

The impression received at a popular level is often that Alzheimer's disease is a single, unitary condition and that it is therefore reasonable to talk in terms of a single, unitary "cause" of the disease, genetic or otherwise. In reality all the evidence would indicate that there is extreme heterogeneity (difference in kind) within what is commonly termed Alzheimer's disease:

"At present no scientist can say with assurance whether Alzheimer's disease (AD) is a single disease, a complex syndrome with many subtypes and varieties of patterns in its manifestations, or many different diseases with similar clusters of symptoms" (Khachaturian 1992).

There is an enormous degree of variation in, for example, age of onset, duration, rate of decline in cognitive function, and extent and type of neurological damage discovered after death. A further distinction can be made between those cases of AD termed "familial" (occurring within families) and those described as "sporadic" (occurring where there is no apparent family history).

Although this heterogeneity is widely acknowledged in scientific circles (Khachaturian 1992), researchers have a regrettable tendency only to "go public" when some new discovery appears for a time to shed light on what is overall a very muddy picture. While a combination of scientific fervour and journalistic licence has often given rise to claims that crucial evidence has been uncovered linking AD to specific "faulty genes" or environmental toxins, the evidence suggests that such a complex range of disorders is very unlikely to have any single or common origin.

Discoveries so far

For the purposes of genetic research two main types of AD are recognised. The first of these is a rare, early-onset, familial form which is claimed to be inherited as an autosomal dominant trait. This means that a person need only inherit one copy of the gene responsible from either of his or her parents in order to develop AD. Because families affected by this autosomal dominant form are rare, however, research opportunities are limited and there are still considerable grounds for scepticism about the data which have emerged to date. Even if it is established that each person affected by this form of AD carries the same gene, it cannot necessarily be concluded that the gene "causes" this form of AD. In order to establish that claim with reasonable certainty it would be necessary to screen large numbers of people in the general population and ascertain that the same gene never occurs in unaffected individuals. This possibility has not, to my knowledge, been considered by any research programme so far.

In all other cases of AD, and these form the great majority, it is generally accepted that the role of genetic factors, if any, is much less significant. What may be inherited is a genetic susceptibility to the condition or, more precisely, to any of the potentially vast number of environmental factors which may be involved in its development.

Very recent research findings appear to bear out this view, focusing attention on the gene responsible for producing a protein called Apolipoprotein E (Apo E). This protein is thought to bind to another (abnormal) protein which is found in the brain of the person with AD. There are three alternative forms of this gene: E2, E3 and E4. Every individual inherits one form of the Apo E gene from each parent, resulting in a combination of any two alleles, eg. E2/E3, E4/E4. It is now thought that inheriting an E4 allele increases the risk of developing AD, whilst the E2 allele appears to give some protection against the condition. It has been emphasised, however, that inheriting an E4 allele, whilst apparently increasing the risk, does not in any sense "cause" AD; nor do the relatively favourable E3 and E2 combinations give any guarantee against it. It is possible to have the "worst" possible E4/E4 allele combination and still not develop AD even in extreme old age, or to have the E2/E3 combination and develop the condition relatively early in life (Roses et al 1994).

This research would seem to indicate that although there may be genetic risk factors involved in AD, they are in no way decisive in terms of who develops AD and who does not. Many other factors affecting the individual after conception must also be involved. The study of such factors is known as "epigenetics" and it entails an understanding of the difference between the "genotype" of an individual (the state of his or genes) which is inherited and fixed at birth, and that person's "phenotype", which is not inherited, but can be understood as the result of a continuous interaction between the genotype and everything that subsequently happens to the person during the course of his or her life – all the features of the physical and social environment in which that person lives (Waddington 1975). In the case of Apo E, for example, a person may have the genotype E4/E4, but the way this is expressed as a phenotype (whether or not the person develops AD and at what age) will depend not only upon this original genotype, but also upon the person's lived experience.

Although this distinction between genotype and phenotype is a basic principle of developmental genetics, researchers in the field of AD rarely do more than pay lip service to it (Rose et al 1984). They may refer in passing to the "possible contribution of epigenetic factors", but they show scant interest in finding out what these may be. It must be clear by now that a purely genetic approach will never be able to give a definitive account of the causes of AD. We might ask why, in that case, such research is progressing apace, while investigation of other possible contributing factors is neglected by comparison, and the actual care of those affected by AD is chronically starved of funding.

Why does genetic research ignore epigenetic factors?

To a large extent, I think the answer to this question lies in the history of genetic theory, beginning with the Darwinian notion of the "survival of the fittest" in the natural world. Darwin's theory was based on the observation that animals produce far more offspring than actually survive. Those which do survive are the strongest and best adapted to the environment and they live to pass on these favourable characteristics to the next generation. Although Darwin's theory of evolution was a major step forward in scientific understanding, it has often been used to support the misguided view that "biology is destiny"; that everything about us is encoded in our genes at birth and cannot be changed.

This kind of thinking has been applied to human societies in some very unfortunate ways. In the late 19th century, for example, "social Darwinists" argued that poverty and ignorance were the result of indiscriminate breeding by people whose inferior characteristics were being allowed to proliferate because they had too many children. Similar ideas informed the "eugenicist" movements which gained strength during the first part of this century, advocating the sterilization of anyone whose "defective genes" might pollute the national stock. Such programmes of racial purification reached their logical conclusion in the gas chambers of Nazi Germany. These are extreme examples, but they illustrate the essential point of the argument: the source of a social problem is located within individual members of society; if people are poor, or ignorant or unhealthy, this is not because there is something wrong with society but because they are afflicted with "defective genes".

The most recent manifestation of this kind of theory – known as "sociobiology" – has taken these beliefs to their extreme, claiming that violence in society, crime, war, and every other social ill can be explained by the fact that we have genes for aggression, selfishness, dislike of strangers and so on (Dawkins 1976). In this view, the properties of individuals are reducible to the properties of their genes and we can understand everything there is to know about human beings by analysing the biochemical properties of the cells which come under the control of these genes. Epigenetic factors are seen as entirely irrelevant.

Few, if any, of the scientists engaged in genetic research into AD would consciously wish to ally themselves with ideas of this nature. No doubt they are motivated as individuals by a genuine desire to alleviate human suffering. Yet it is still the case that their training and the methods they use originate from a tradition of determinist and reductionist theory, and this can often lead to a kind of tunnel vision in which the real, living, interacting person is barely considered. In modern molecular genetics there is an almost exclusive concentration on developing increasingly sophisticated methods for studying the individual genotype and very little consideration is given to the way its phenotypic expression may be influenced by, for example, living in a society where ageing is often accompanied by alienation, isolation and material deprivation.

We know from the many "sporadic" cases which develop where there is no family history that the role of epigenetic factors in AD must be very significant. Although we may not know as yet what all these factors are, there seems every reason to believe that anything which has a bearing on physical and mental health will play a large part – not only in determining who develops AD and who does not – but also on the course the condition follows in those who do succumb to it. This does not mean, however, that we should reject the idea that genetic factors play any part at all in the development of AD and look instead for solely environmental causes. Instead we need to aim for an understanding of the way many different factors constantly in interaction with each other can contribute to the onset and course of AD.

How do genetic and environmental factors interact?

A simple way of illustrating this point is to use the example of eye colour – an inherited trait which is often used to demonstrate genetic transmission and which most people remember from school. The gene for brown eyes is dominant over the genes for any other eye colour and a child need only inherit one copy of this gene from either parent in order to have brown eyes. The fact that the child has inherited the genotype for brown eyes from the parent does not mean,

however, that there is any one-to-one correspondence between the eye colour of parent and child. In fact no two pairs of eyes can ever be identical in colour or in any other respect. The phenotype will always be different from the genotype even when a dominant gene is involved.

We are also told that, through the process of natural selection, the gene for brown eyes has become dominant because brown eyes are stronger than eyes of any other colour, and that brown-eyed people are therefore less likely to suffer from defective vision. However, although there may be general truth in the claim that inheriting the gene for brown eyes is advantageous, this is not necessarily true at the phenotypic level. The brown eyes of a malnourished Somalian refugee with cataracts are clearly not stronger than the blue eyes of a well-fed Swiss banker; and even if the Swiss banker does have defective eyesight this can easily be corrected by wearing spectacles. Even in the apparently trivial case of eye colour then, we can see that a genotypic advantage can be cancelled out by the lived experience of the individual, just as a genotypic disadvantage can be enhanced by a beneficial environment.

If we now move on to consider the way genetic and environmental factors interact in AD, the picture should have become somewhat clearer. Firstly, we can see that even if it were to be established beyond doubt that some cases of AD are inherited by means of a dominant gene in the same way as eye colour, there would still be a limit to what genetics could tell us, because the phenotype of the individual is always unique. It would not be possible to infer anything definite about age of onset or rate of decline in an individual by knowing his or her genotype. Just as no two pairs of eyes could ever be identical in colour, no two cases of AD will ever follow exactly the same course.

The explanation for these differences must lie somewhere outside the genotype, in the interaction between the person and every aspect of his or her environment from the moment of conception onwards. Nor do these environmental factors simply "pile up" on top of the original genotype; they interact with it, so that a new phenotype is constantly in the process of creation. It is this process of interaction which can tip the balance either way in relation to which individual develops AD and which does not.

Moreover, even in those cases where AD does develop, the phenotype will continue to change and the fact that this is a "degenerative" condition does not necessarily mean that the direction of change must be for the worse. In the example of the Somalian refugee above, we can see that good food, a safe place to feel at home, and an operation to remove cataracts would change the situation enormously. Such practical changes can also make an enormous difference to the person with AD, working to lessen the effect of an underlying deterioration. Where it is also possible to offer improved social relationships, opportunities for growth, and recognition of personhood there are considerable grounds for optimism that the condition can be reversed to a significant extent.

For the person with AD, in fact, the implications for care are exactly the same whether the condition is inherited or not, but for family members the question of heritability will inevitably have greater significance. We also need to consider the question of genetic screening for AD, and the potential of genetic research in developing a treatment or cure.

Will genetic research lead to a cure for AD?

To a large extent genetics has never been "about" treating individuals. Its aim, baldly stated, has been to identify unfavourable genotypes in the population and remove them by one means or another. Although there are occasional hints that a new discovery about the genetic basis of AD may lead to a cure at some point in the future, it does not appear that this is even a remote possibility at present. Current research is leading in the direction of developing predictive and diagnostic tests for AD, rather than towards a cure.

The ethical implications of testing for a condition where there is no treatment or cure are profound and complex. In those cases of AD which are held to be autosomally dominant, a test would reveal either the presence or the absence of the dominant gene, and would therefore, in theory, constitute a definite prediction for the condition, either positive or negative. However, unless it is established beyond doubt that the dominant gene in question causes AD in every case there is a serious risk that people may be misinformed by such a test. The fear and anxiety arising from a positive test may arguably be a more significant risk factor for AD than the actual presence of the dominant gene itself.

In all other cases, moreover, all that a test would reveal would be a greater or lesser degree of susceptibility to the condition which would have little, if any, value to the person concerned. The Apo E genotype, for example, can be identified by a simple blood test, and there is a possibility that this may become widely available in the near future, but as we have already seen, knowing the genotype would give an individual no useful information about his or her true likelihood of developing AD.

Unfortunately, the pursuit of genes often appears to take on its own peculiar logic, in which the identification of a genetic cause is seen somehow as an end in itself, almost as though the gene might have the recipe for a cure engraved upon it. For example, under a chapter subheading "Knowledge of the genome will aid the fight against the disease", the geneticist James Watson complains: "Getting the gene(s) for Alzheimer's disease, however, may be very difficult, in part because family histories with accurate diagnoses are hard to get. Many of those with the gene will be missed, since they will die of another disease before they come down with Alzheimer's disease" (Watson 1993).

Watson's chapter makes no reference at all to how "getting the genes" actually will "aid the fight against the disease", and the overall impression gained is that it is pretty inconsiderate for people to die with their genes still "un-got".

In reality, cures have not developed from discovering genetic causes. In fact the progress of medicine throughout history has not on the whole depended on discovering "causes" at all. All the major diseases of the past, tuberculosis is one example, were on the decline long before their causes were understood simply because of improved living conditions, and "medicine remains, despite all the talk...essentially an empirical process in which one does what works" (Lewontin 1993).

The case of Huntington's disease can be used to illustrate what is likely to happen when predictive tests become available. Huntington's disease is an incurable, hereditary, degenerative disorder of the nervous system whose symptoms usually develop when the affected person is in his or her 40s. Pre-symptomatic testing for Huntington's disease is already available, and although it is only 95 per cent accurate it has recently been suggested that it should be made compulsory. It has also been claimed that it would be possible to eradicate the condition in one generation by sampling genetic material from all foetuses conceived by people with the disease, and aborting all those that carried the genetic marker for Huntington's. In fact nothing of any positive benefit to sufferers from Huntington's disease has emerged from genetic research into the condition, leading one commentator to observe that about all the new genetics can offer such a person is to wish they had never been born (Spallone 1992).

There is little in this headlong pursuit to discover and eliminate genes at any cost which offers hope or reassurance to the family of a person with AD. What can be done to improve this situation?

Genetic research and the new culture of dementia care

We can see that there is a pressing need at the present time for clear, constructive and humanely-offered information about the genetic aspects of AD, which takes as its central concerns the needs of those directly affected – the person with AD and their family. This must be given priority over the mere accumulation of scientific knowledge for its own sake. Recognising this is an important aspect of the transition from the old culture of dementia care to the new for two major reasons.

Firstly, the old culture has been marked by a deference toward experts as the source of all knowledge. As "experts", these professionals are often reluctant to make any public admission of doubt. Also, in many cases the medical training of doctors, particularly if it was received some time ago, will not have equipped them to engage on a human level with people in distress, a situation which they may experience as enormously threatening.

Confronted by the kinds of questions family members will often ask when someone they love begins to dement, therefore, doctors will often fall back on impersonal, biological explanations which liken the condition to some form of mechanical breakdown. Genetic explanations are very likely to be seized upon because they carry implications of inevitability which may ease the doctor's feeling of helplessness at being unable to offer any treatment or cure.

However, this kind of response does not recognise the need for comfort and reassurance implicit in the questions likely to be asked. When someone asks, for example, "Why does my mother sometimes not recognise me?", this is obviously not the same kind of question as, "Why is my television set not working?", and it does not deserve the response that there is just some kind of fault in the wiring, or a defect in the brain which can be traced back to a genetic cause. Similarly, when a family member asks about his or her own risk of inheriting AD, what is needed is informed and supportive counselling, not a statistical estimate of probability.

The new culture of dementia care will need to encourage professionals to drop their masks of "expertise", and admit the feelings of doubt and inadequacy which they will inevitably feel at times; it will need to encourage them to share in the distress and fear experienced by those with AD and their families, and to answer their questions in a way which is sensitive to the needs which are being expressed.

Secondly, the new culture of dementia care will demand a rethinking of attitudes toward ageing and disability. The theories which have informed much of the genetic research to date have been based on the marginalisation of those most in need, rather than the acceptance and inclusion they deserve. This kind of thinking derives from a long tradition of representing mental distress and confusion as some form of malignancy within the individual. Centuries ago, the explanation used to be "possession by devils". Today it often seems that "possession by genes" has been substituted for this notion. Increasingly, the impression is given that the body is merely a temporary receptacle for the genes which use it as an instrument in order to reproduce and then move on. Genes are seen as somehow endowed with a consciousness which is superior to that of the person who houses them, and once the genes have succeeded in proliferating they have no further use for the body which can be left to die a helpless and undignified death. We are, in the words of the sociobiologist Richard Dawkins, "mere lumbering robots...whose genes created us body and mind" (Dawkins 1976). In this view of humanity there is clearly no potential for acceptance and affirmation of the person with AD. In fact the neurozoologist, Kirkwood, has gone so far as to develop a "disposable soma (or body) theory" of Alzheimer's disease in which the person is reduced to little more than a derelict and decaying building whose occupants have moved out (report in *The Independent*, 1992).

It hardly needs saying that this kind of thinking has no place in the new culture of dementia care. However, whilst it may be the case that some scientists are so devoted to these dehumanising and mechanistic notions as to be beyond reform, there will be many more who will be open to new ways of thinking. We need to argue wherever possible for a new, more humane form of biomedical science which has clear, practical, human outcomes – a science which delivers the means actually to help people. And in the meantime we need to keep hold of our "reasonable scepticism" and continue to question the motives and methods of current scientific research.

References

Dawkins R (1976) *The Selfish Gene*. Oxford University Press, Oxford.

Khachaturian Z. S. (1992) *Heterogeneity of Alzheimer's Disease*. Springer-Verlag, Berlin.

Lewontin R (1993) *The Doctrine of DNA*. Penguin, London.

Rose S, Kamin L, Lewontin R (1984) *Not in Our Genes*. Pelican, Harmondsworth.

Roses AD, Strittmatter W J, Pericak-Vance MA, Corder EH, Saunders AM, Schmechel DE. Letter to *The Lancet*, 18th June, 1994.

Spallone P (1992) *Generation Games*. The Women's Press, London

The Independent "Effects of age on body linked to role of genes". News report 27th March, 1992.

Waddington CH (1975) *The Evolution of an Evolutionist*. Edinburgh University Press, Edinburgh.

Watson J (1993). "The human genome initiative". In *Genetics and Society* Holland B, Charalambos K, (eds) Addison-Wesley, Wokingham.

CHAPTER
TEN

Support through human contact for family carers

ERROLYN BRUCE

Dementia care is not easy. Family carers need other people to understand the difficulties, appreciate their efforts and encourage them to face up to the issues at the heart of caring. Support means giving time to carers as they struggle to make sense of dementia.

*T*here are many different ways to support family carers (1). One kind of support is practical help. It is absolutely essential, because it relieves carers of some of their many tasks, and gives them a little time to attend to things they could not otherwise do. Respite care, day care, home care and sitting services are examples of practical help – effectively substitute care – often experienced by carers as a lifeline. However, the focus of this chapter is not on support to carers through practical help and periodic relief from caring tasks, but on support through human contact, or social support. I shall argue that this form of support is of great value, but must stress that it should not be seen as a substitute for practical help, or a device for cutting the costs of services.

It is not easy to come to terms with the fact that someone close to you has dementia, and to accept all that this means for you and for the person concerned. Faced with this unpleasant reality, a person creates his or her own understanding of the situation. Typically this begins as an inconsistent and shifting account, and gradually becomes a more coherent story. The story will evolve as the situation changes and as new information is acquired.

Support through human contact can enable people's understandings to evolve so that they work well, both for the carer and for the person they are looking after. When the person cared for has been a main source of support for the carer in the past, this support must come from other relationships. However, dealing with dementia is an out of the ordinary experience and family relationships and other friendships may not be able to meet a carer's needs fully. Indeed, at times they can be an added source of stress. People familiar with dementia but relatively detached from the particular sufferer can play an important part in providing support.

Support through human contact can occur in many different contexts: as a by-product of providing practical help, in passing from an understanding professional or formally in support groups, counselling, befriending and so on. In this chapter I shall look at three aspects of providing this type of support that are common to all settings: firstly, the ways in which support through human contact can be helpful; secondly, points to consider when making support appropriate and thirdly, some of the key issues which it is necessary (but not always easy) for carers to face. Comments in italics are from carers who have been through our Focus on Dementia programme (2).

Does it help? Taking a broader view of support

You get a whole new approach to things instead of being overwhelmed by the whole situation – Betty Waters

Research on carers' support groups has not always shown them to be particularly effective in reducing stress as measured by psychological tests. Perhaps this is not surprising since the source of stress – someone close to you having an incurable illness and an ongoing need for care – is not changed by joining a group.

However, there are other reasons for extending support to carers than merely attempting to reduce stress. Not only do participants in groups speak highly of them and feel that the experience was worthwhile, but also the offer of support to carers is an essential strand of expressing social responsibility for personal misfortune, rather than leaving individuals in trouble to fend for themselves (Toseland 1989, Abel 1990). Taking this broader view of the purpose of carers' support, there are ways in which it can be helpful regardless of whether it succeeds in reducing stress.

---

1. People with dementia who live in the community are looked after by a wide variety of different people. For simplicity I refer to this diverse group of people as "family carers" or just "carers", though some are not family and many would not call themselves carers. Despite the common threads running through the experience of caring, it is important to recognise that social divisions – eg gender, generation, ethnicity, class – and other factors – eg co-residence, relationship history, family context – make the experience very different for different people.
2. I am indebted to David Coates for this material. He is evaluating the Focus on Dementia programme and most of these comments are taken from his interviews with carers. Names have been changed.

Acknowledging the challenge

Support for carers acknowledges the huge challenge of caring. It is not an ideal situation when a person's life is subsumed to another person's needs and daily care. Responses to carers are often determined by gender. Whereas men who take on this role may be praised and admired, the far larger numbers of women involved in caring are commonly seen to be just doing their duty (Rose and Bruce 1984). Both men and women complain that people do not understand what caring is like. Carers whatever their gender need understanding and appreciation of what they do.

Countering abandonment

Carers frequently experience isolation and abandonment (Alzheimer's Disease Society 1993). Elderly people looking after a spouse with dementia often feel that everyone else is having a good time enjoying an active retirement while all their plans have been shattered. Daughters typically lose status and income as result of leaving work, and are strung between the conflicting needs of different generations (Brody 1981). Offering support to carers helps to combat the experience of being left alone with one's personal misfortune, and communicates our willingness to walk alongside, however briefly.

It's just that you're not on your own, that's the main thing – Dulcie Haywood
That's a tremendous thing, that we don't feel alone any more – Betty Waters

Creating a place of understanding

It is not always socially acceptable to talk about illnesses and bodily functions. The day to day dilemmas of caring don't really fit into polite neighbourly exchanges, and carers may want to protect the dignity of the person they care for in their immediate social world. Carers' support creates a setting where caring is the norm and it is socially acceptable to discuss the details of the process. Where carers meet in a group, this effect is enhanced and many people find it empowering to exchange experiences with others in similar situations.

I've been able to say things that I wouldn't say to anyone actually, outside the group…it's easier to talk to someone who kinda knows what you're talking about – Leila Browning

Recognising difficult feelings

Caring is characterised by difficult feelings. The central paradox for many carers is that they both want and do not want to be a carer. Though trapped, and unable to live life as they want, exhausted and worried about their own health, carers know that the person they look after is better off at home and they want the best for them. Many everyday relationships cannot accommodate a perpetual rollercoaster of emotion. Carers' support provides a context in which feelings can be expressed, and mixed feelings and inconsistency are acceptable. Living with loss, and fears about the future and about death can be explored.

You bring a lot of things out that's in the back of your mind that you don't really think's there until somebody else starts discussing it – Dulcie Haywood
You've really to examine your feelings and that's good because you tend not to do that, be busy with everyday things – Betty Waters

Supporting learning

Caring demands new skills and the ability find out about a changing situation. Carers learn their role through performing it, but carers' support can make the learning process smoother. People often say "if only I'd known about that sooner". Support increases the chances that carers find out what they need when they need it, and are better prepared to accept successive changes. When a person is under stress, learning about things relating to the cause of stress is specially challenging. Difficult feelings may need to be faced before information can be taken in, or before knowledge can be acted upon. Confidence enhances learning so it is helpful to acknowledge carers' existing skills and expertise.

Making sure support is appropriate

There are many good ways to offer support to suit different people and circumstances. However, whether the support offered is a brief intervention or ongoing, whether to an individual or to a group, it is important to make sure that it is appropriate. The following factors are things which many carers say are important to them, and help to make support really supportive.

Respect for expertise, and empowerment

Carers have detailed specialist knowledge about the course of dementia in their particular person. They may also build up considerable knowledge of local services and the financial aspects of caring. Despite this, carers are at risk of feeling crushed by their situation. Loss of confidence, resignation and poor emotional well-being are reported in many studies (Parker 1985).

On the other hand many people survive caring, and although they would never have chosen the experience, do feel better able to face up to adversity as a result. In Focus on Dementia we present a simple model of survival, to give hope and to suggest that it is possible for any ordinary person to weather caring, not just wonderful men and superwomen. In groups, carers have the opportunity to help one another. They can give as well as receive support, which can be empowering. However, careful facilitation is needed to ensure that everyone accepts that dementia can be very different for different people and that each person has to form their own interpretation of what is happening in their own case.

I said "we've got a lot to give to this"... you become more aware of what you can do for other people – Richard Oldroyd

The problem of information overload

There is a vast amount of written information available to carers about different aspects of caring and how to find and use services. Some people respond to the caring situation by reading everything they can find, but most people do not want to acquire a vast body of knowledge about the subject. They do, however, want to know what they need to know when they need to use it. This can be problematic in a situation where everything from brain science to local day care provision is changing. Perhaps the most useful information is that which helps people to find out where, or who, to go to when the time comes.

I'm not very good at books – I mean converting what was written in the book to doing it – Richard Oldroyd

Time for problems of the moment

Carers typically have their patience stretched to its limits many times a week, if not many times a day. Against the backdrop of long-running concerns about the person they look after, there are often set a number of immediate problems or irritations which need airing. Many carers have a lot to put up with, and may benefit from a chance to talk about small things, and indeed may need to "empty their top drawer" to be able to concentrate on other matters. Appropriate carers' support needs to put carers' experiences at the centre, and allow time for immediate problems.

There was room for people to say what they wanted to say...if somebody brought up something then they'd follow it up – Maria Semenec

The value of facing fears

Carers' support must balance the need to be prepared for the future against the risk of fuelling anxieties about the gloomy possibilities that it may hold. For many people it is possible to listen to the experiences of others without being alarmed by the thought of what they may have to deal with. Hearing about the experiences of people who have been caring for longer than themselves is for many people a good way to take in knowledge about things they hope will not happen, but might.

It takes out the fear of what's going to happen...you can sort of prepare yourself for it a bit – Maria Semenec

They were happier after thinking about it because it got over the bogey that one must think about it – Richard Oldroyd.

Awareness of suppressed issues

In any situation there are some things that are hard to discuss. A mixed sex group may avoid discussions of sexual feelings. A support group run by staff from a day care centre feel unable to discuss the quality of care at the centre. It is probably impossible to create the circumstances under which any topic feels possible to everyone, but it is useful to be aware of the limitations of particular situations. Sometimes inviting people to discuss a sticky topic is enough to make it possible.

The need for help

The task overload experienced by carers means that sometimes what they really need is for someone else to get something sorted out for them. Carers constantly have to leave tasks undone, because one person just cannot manage everything. On occasions carers in groups will offer to do things for each other. It may also be appropriate for facilitators to do things for people. Help of this kind is not disempowering if the carer remains in control of what is done.

I've got so much on sometimes I just long for a Georgette Heyer hero to come charging in and sort it all out for me...take it off my hands – Michelle Slater

You've got organisers who will find things out for you – Betty Waters

Finding ways to create movement

Carers can get stuck in a state of gloomy resignation. Carers' support needs to find ways to help people accept the unchangeable aspects of their situation, and to be able to give enough challenge to create movement and change. Some things cannot be changed, but people can change how they feel about them. Humour can have a very powerful effect. Seeing the funny side of tragic events helps to make them less overwhelming

It got me out of my shell...I mean I've started to come out of a very dark hole...I couldn't have done it without the group – Richard Oldroyd

At the heart of caring

"They took any subject and made it manageable .... They chewed at it until, softened, it yielded, like blubber or leather to their understanding. They went over it repeatedly until it weakened and gave in and became part of them. Tragedy, disaster: they moulded them into small, digestible portions." (From *Daughters of the House* by Michèle Roberts, Virago 1992.)

Taking the experience of dementia caring and reducing it to small digestible portions is the essence of carers' support. It entails working with the immediate day to day problems that people are having, but also facing up to some issues which lie at the heart of the caring experience. The nature of the understanding that people develop is very important: "old culture" understandings of dementia are not always conducive to enhancing the quality of life either for people with dementia, or for their carers.

The meaning of dementia

A diagnosis of dementia is hard to accept, and understanding of what is entailed goes beyond the bare facts of the dementing illnesses, though these are important. Going over the process of diagnosis and making sense of what has happened since can help people to accept the unpalatable reality that the person they look after will not recover.

Hope lies in making the crucial distinction between the fact that dementia is incurable and the belief that nothing can be done for a person with dementia. Despite incurability, there are ways to enable people who suffer from dementia get the best out of their lives, despite the disabling effects of their illness. Carers are all different, and each individual needs to explore the meaning of dementia in their own life.

Dealing with feelings; living with loss

Caring inevitably throws up difficult, and usually mixed, feelings. Carers' support is an opportunity for carers to identify and express their feelings and realise that dealing with difficult feelings is an inevitable and recurring part of looking after someone with dementia. As well as their own feelings carers also have to recognise and understand the difficult feelings of the person with dementia. In particular, both are living with loss, the process of grieving is woven into their daily lives, and will shape their reactions to events. Both may find comfort in past memories, and in making the most of small pleasures of the moment. People with dementia may benefit from finding some words to describe what is happening to them.

Tangled lives – the power of de-centering

Caring brings two lives into closer proximity than before, and two sets of needs and interests can become tangled together. De-centering means that the carer looks at the situation from the viewpoint of the person with dementia as well as from their own perspective. Guessing how things feel for the person with dementia is a powerful way to disentangle the complexities of the situation, and to become clearer about those things that can be changed and those that cannot. It is also the first step to learning to re-frame problems.

Sometimes re-framing a problem suggests a course of action which will lead to the problem going away; at other times it makes it clear that there is no way to remove the problem, but may help the carer to become more able to live with it. When carers are able to separate their own needs from those of the person they look after and to accept that there are conflicts of interest, they are better able to find flexible solutions to the problems of dependency. The situation they are in is not ideal. Neither person can have exactly what they need or want, but in each circumstance a best compromise needs to be found.

Facing the future

Some people like to plan for every eventuality, whereas others prefer to deal with events as they arise. When looking after someone with dementia, some things are predictable. If the person with dementia is very dependent on their carer, then it is certain that should the carer be killed in an accident or taken into hospital, there will be a crisis. If the carer wishes to have some control over what happens should such a crisis occur, then some planning and preparation is necessary.

In most cases, however, it is highly likely that the person with dementia will die before their carer. Adjusting to this final bereavement may be helped by giving the carers the opportunity to explore their feelings about it in advance.

Social life and social support

While there is evidence for social support as a factor in health and well-being (Cohen & Syme 1985), there is little doubt that social contacts can be both vital to well-being and the cause of great distress. Keeping up a satisfying social life as a carer – and arranging one for the person with dementia – can be difficult. Family members, friends and neighbours do not always react to dementia in a helpful way. Complex family dynamics can combine with the difficulties caused by dementia to make things very tricky for carers.

Pausing to consider the feelings that lie behind people's reactions, along with some assertiveness, can help carers to maintain worthwhile relationships, despite the fact that some of the people important to them may have negative responses to dementia. New activities and new friends may be needed to fill the gap left when pursuits enjoyed in the past are given up, and people with whom the problems of caring can be aired may need to be found.

Finding and using sources of help

Accepting outside help can be a difficult step, particularly for spouses caring for a partner (Thornton 1989). It can be difficult to find out what help is available, but often there are further problems when it comes to using the services on offer. Carers need to accept that other people will care for their person differently from the way they do, and that there may be advantages as well as disadvantages to these differences.

On the other hand the quality of care provided to

people with dementia is not always as high as it should be, and they may be faced with difficult decisions such as whether to continue using a particular service, and if so, how to encourage service providers to meet their friend or relative's needs.

Fitting services into one's life is often difficult, and there are usually costs as well as benefits. For example a sitter coming to look after someone at home may suit the person with dementia and give the carer valuable time off but also leave her feeling that their home has been invaded. Exploring these issues is helpful, both in enabling carers to start using the services that they need, and in coming to terms with mixed feelings about continuing to use them.

An essential part of the new culture

It's like having your mother at the back of you...it's been a god-send to me...it's given me a lot of confidence – Dulcie Haywood

Carers themselves can be quite clear about what they find supportive, and what they do not. People working in the field of dementia care need to listen to what they have to say, and to try to offer support in many different forms to suit different tastes and circumstances. We need to reach out to all carers and convey the message that their efforts are appreciated, and that they are not alone. Certainly they deserve recognition.

I always felt better when I came out. I don't know why, it just seemed to give me a lift – Maggie Greenwood

A further intriguing possibility is that carers' support could also benefit people with dementia. There is as yet no hard evidence for this, but comments like these certainly lead us to consider the extent to which a better supported carer will provide a better quality of care to their person with dementia:

If I hadn't had the group, either my mum wouldn't have been here now or I'd have been in hospital with a nervous breakdown, really – Leila Browning

I think I'm happier with her...I can see that she's still the person I've been with for so many years. Behind everything, the same person...I'm glad to go and see her now, whereas before, I had to go and see her – Richard Oldroyd

There is evidence that social support in other contexts can have far-reaching effects (3), and the possibility that the provision of appropriate support to carers could benefit the people they care for as well as carers themselves gives further reason to see carers' support as an essential part of the new culture of dementia care.

References

Abel EK (1990) Informal care for the disabled elderly: a critique of recent literature. *Research on Aging* **12** 139-157.

Alzheimer's Disease Society (1993) *Deprivation and Dementia.*

Brody EM (1981) "Women in the middle" and family help to older people. *The Gerontologist* **21(5)**.

Cohen S & Syme SL eds (1985) *Social Support and Health.* Academic Press, London.

Parker G (1985) With due care and attention: a review of research on informal care. *Occasional Paper No 2,* Family Policy Studies Centre, London.

Rose H and Bruce E (forthcoming) "Mutual care but differential esteem" in Arber S and Ginn J (eds) *Connecting Gender and Ageing* (working title), Open University Press.

Toseland RW and Rossiter CM (1989) Group interventions to support family caregivers: a review and analysis. *The Gerontologist* **29** 438-448.

Thornton P (1989) The needs of elderly spouse carers: a neglected research issue. *Generations* **10** 15-19.

3. For example, among women who had had a previous low birth-weight baby those who received support during a subsequent pregnancy had heavier babies who were healthier and needed fewer visits to the doctor during their first year of life than the babies of those women who had standard NHS care during pregnancy. Oakley A (1988) Is social support good for the health of mothers and babies? *Journal of Reproductive and Infant Psychology* **6** 3-21.

CHAPTER ELEVEN | Backs to the wall? Day care within the new culture

PAUL CUNNINGHAM
JANE KESTERTON

Embracing the ideas and practice of the new culture led to a radical review of day centre services for individuals with dementia. This chapter describes five areas where change was achieved and brought great benefits, including greatly increased involvement of prime carers in care planning, and the demolition of barriers between "us" (staff) and "them".

*A*lthough some day care places have been available to individuals with dementia since the dawn of day care provision for older people, day care facilities designed especially for them, and their carers, are a relatively modern phenomenon. Early provision was offered within integrated centres for "the elderly" where basic personal care was provided, together with a hot meal and transport to and from the centre. Those individuals who did not fit the service provided, or became a problem, were prevented from attending, and as there was no alternative provision stayed at home with their carers.

The introduction of "special" days for individuals with dementia led to some degree of provision – a respite service for carers and containment for the service users. This service was frequently only available one day a week at each centre, but it was a start. Seven day care in a specialist centre followed, but the care remained very much respite based, with the focus on carers as service users, not the individuals with dementia.

The new culture of dementia care, and the person-centred approach, has enabled us to begin to create a balance between the support we offer to carers through respite, and the way in which we meet the individual care needs of the person with dementia. We are now enabled to work *with* the prime carers (1) rather than *for* them, to provide the type of care both they and the person they care for wish to receive.

The new culture has led us to review care practice within our day centres for individuals with dementia so radically that it is impossible for us to cover all the changes within this chapter. We have chosen to look at

five areas we identified as offering opportunities for change, where we were able to introduce the new culture and improve the service we offered. Finally in this chapter we will look at some of the unresolved issues in establishing the new culture in day care.

Admission to day care

In the old culture we inherited, there was little emphasis on the admission process of a person with dementia into a day care setting. Often the criteria for admission consisted of a planned day visit during which the centre staff would "assess" whether or not they could manage the person with dementia. The idea would be for the person to fit into the service, arriving and departing at set times, joining in the activities provided and sharing the same social graces as the other persons receiving the service. A person with dementia who did not "fit in" would be deemed too difficult to manage and therefore unsuitable for placement.

Through providing a specialist day care service for older people with dementia, a more humanistic approach has been adopted. Now we view each prospective service user as a human being with an individual history, biography, likes, dislikes and expectations for the future. In other words, we look at the person behind the dementia. This approach ensures, through domiciliary visits, that the person with dementia is given information about the service and is given the opportunity to discuss with a staff member the care they require in an environment in which they are comfortable.

A major improvement brought about by this approach is the contribution made by prime carers at a very early stage of care planning, as advocates for the person they care for and advisers in the setting up of appropriate resources. Both the prime carers and the person with dementia are then invited to visit the centre in order for them to assess whether the service is appropriate to their needs. During this visit the centre staff, through observation and further discussion, are able to ascertain the individual requirements of the prospective service user. While the centre staff may not be able to commit themselves to

---

1. I have used the term "prime carers" because in my experience the main carer of a day centre service user is often not a member of their family but a friend or neighbour.

meeting all these needs immediately, they will provide a base from which to move forward and develop a programme of accessible appropriate care.

We see this initial introductory process as the start of a sharing relationship between the centre staff and the prime carers, promoting a positive approach to working together to provide care for the person with dementia. The prime carers may be family, close friends or neighbours and the sharing of care with them has proved to be a dynamic process where paid and unpaid carers provide each other with information and support to enhance the quality of life for the person with dementia. We hope that the time of unpaid carers being given the cold shoulder, as not qualified to intervene with day centre care, is over now that a new more informed culture of dementia care has come into being.

Recognition and support: carers in the new culture

In the past, the caring professions have worked hard to promote their own power and status, particularly through the use of jargon, abbreviation and unnecessarily long words. They projected an idealistic image of themselves as having far-reaching knowledge and skills which the unpaid carer could not hope to attain. The professionals place themselves in an advisory role in relation to the carers, proffering solutions to problems never identified and insight into behaviours never observed. This behaviour has been further reinforced by day centres where prime carers are made to feel that staff have specialised skills that they do not possess. A feeling of inferiority manifests itself leaving the unpaid carers isolated and hopeless; these carers then withdraw from the centre and their valuable input is lost.

Within the new culture of dementia care we attempt to include all carers in the centre activities so that they may become, should they wish to, fully involved in the world of those for whom they care.

A monthly Carers' Group provides a forum for exchanging information and advice, learning relaxation techniques, catching up on the latest developments, checking out on benefits or generally having a good gossip. The group sets the agenda, arranges speakers, plans activities and the centre staff offer support and assistance as required. The meetings take place within the day centre so that all carers can become involved. The centre staff are on hand to care for the persons with dementia who accompany their carers.

Joint activities organised by the centre have included a very successful restaurant visit for Christmas, involving carers, service users and staff, enabling one couple who had not danced together for years to take to the floor. At a summer barbeque the back-handed compliment – "You could almost believe there was nothing wrong with

them" – was welcomed by one of the carers.

We try to be flexible with our approach to carers' needs regarding opening/closing hours and requests for odd additional days, to allow the prime carers to lead less restricted lives. We do try to listen and we have learned from experience that we are dependent on the carers to give us help and advice with our work. They know the person with dementia far more intimately than we ever will. At least, the new culture welcomes unpaid carers; we do at our centre, but there is still a long way to go. We know that we can still appear offhand and busy but we hope that we can be forgiven – we are trying to change.

Demolishing the barriers between "us" and "them"

The barriers that we create between ourselves as staff and the persons who use our service became obvious from a dementia care mapping exercise carried out in the centre. (The method of this exercise is outlined in chapter 15.) The analysis of the data collected indicated that there was little interaction between staff and service users. Considering this we became aware of an unspoken assumption: "we" (the staff) are of course sound of mind and unimpaired, whereas "they" (the users) are people with dementia and the ones who cause the problems. But we are all human beings, so why were there barriers between us that prevented interaction? Were we going to catch dementia by using the same crockery, sitting on the same chair or using the same toilets? We decided that we did not need the barriers so we looked for ways to dismantle them.

One area where we felt this was possible was identified during another mapping exercise. Here we found that centre users spent 25 per cent of their time eating and drinking, but they were not necessarily experiencing any great degree of well-being during this activity. We felt that we could improve this situation by encouraging the centre staff to sit and take their meals with the service users. Free meals for the staff were negotiated and these staff became participants instead of supervisors.

The results were excellent. The member of staff at each table not only promoted appropriate eating skills but encouraged conversation and general interaction during the meal. This was the first move towards breaking down the barriers between "us" and "them". It also provided an ideal opportunity for validation and reminiscence therapy, as well as reality orientation, without having to formalise these activities under those names. We participated in their world instead of imposing our world on them.

Having developed this new culture, which has its roots in the person-centred approach, we built on it. Our staff have become participants instead of supervisors in many areas including exercise groups, media groups and discussions. This may not sound particularly innovative, but as previous training for working with individuals with dementia has consisted primarily of methods of containment followed by further training on management of the subsequent violence and aggression, it was in fact a giant step forward. It was as if we had been arming ourselves against the marauding masses. However, the masses were not marauding; they looked like ordinary human beings. And so we now treat them as we would our other friends.

To our shame, the mapping exercise had also shown that few toilet visits took place. Those who required assistance were taken or reminded but on one particular day nobody else visited the toilet at all. We started reminding everyone where the toilets were when they arrived and at intervals during the day. Our personal belief is that if toilets are good enough for service users then they are good enough for the staff. The next step in the barrier demolition programme is for the staff, when making their own toilet visits, to check with service users to see if they wish to go. This is particularly relevant as many prime carers told us that the person they care for always accompanies them to the toilet. As this initiative takes effect, we are sure continence difficulties will be greatly reduced.

One good outcome of the new culture of dementia care in day centres is that it allows the staff to participate and the persons with dementia to choose not to. We will carry on in this direction.

Recognising the person

In the section above we have used two areas to illustrate the way in which we are trying to break down the barriers. Perhaps the best way to achieve this is to recognise the person; we have not forgotten the root of the new culture – personhood. We too recognise, as did Oliver Stone in his screenplay of Oliver Sachs book "Awakenings" that:

Human spirit is more powerful than any drug and that is what needs to be nourished. Work, play, family, friendship, these are the things that matter. This is what we had forgotten – the simplest things.
(Stone 1992)

The person-centred approach does not overlook the simple things. It identifies them and in doing so nourishes the human spirit so that a person with dementia can lead the full and fulfilling life to which they have a right. We support this by the building up of a user profile with the assistance of the service user, prime carer, centre staff and any significant others who play a role in the life of the person with dementia.

The profile begins from the first time the person and their carer have contact with the centre, and slowly builds up into a detailed picture of the person. We include the names of those important to that person, alive and dead, their personal likes and dislikes, favourite foods and drinks, and dietary needs, especially those relating to health and religious requirements. Also included are any records from childhood, schooldays, or previous employment and hobbies or areas of particular interest – anything that will identify that person as an individual.

As long as we see service users as a homogenous group we will never deliver appropriate care; the "they" label is almost as difficult to dispose of as the "us" and "them" barrier. This barrier is the key to all of the malignant social psychology that Tom Kitwood has detailed, and which is such a strong feature of the old culture of care (Kitwood 1990).

Within our centres we are attempting to try and understand and accept the service users' feelings. This will allow individuals to do things for themselves according to their capabilities. We will not always assume that we must take control, which can result in these adults being treated like children. We try to meet each individual at whatever level we can engage in real contact, whether through speech, touch or simple eye contact. We try to validate and not dismiss each person's feelings although they may be alien to us.

We also try to interpret the meaning behind the person's words and actions even if at first their sense is doubtful. This is why it is so important to build up a profile of each individual. With this aid it is often possible to interpret otherwise unintelligible language, if we put it within the context of the person's own terms of reference.

Above all we try to make time for people and go through the day at an appropriate pace for each individual. This can often mean that each person is doing a different thing at a different time, with the consequent difficulties this brings for staff members who must attempt to co-ordinate these activities. We constantly remind ourselves and our staff to address persons with dementia by their preferred name and always to explain exactly what is about to happen.

We are far from perfect, and we do make mistakes, However these mistakes show that we are human and bring to our caring our own emotions and feelings. We need to be able to express our emotions freely within the care environment to enable persons with dementia to have the freedom to do the same.

The care environment

Good care involves not only what occurs at an interpersonal level, but also the actual physical environment. We would not dispute that excellent care may be offered in a poor environment, but a little thought led us to create more appropriate surroundings without too much effort. We began to reflect on the possibility that we are disabling persons with dementia by not providing the environment in which they could flourish. Out of season magazines, incorrect calendars and unreliable wall clocks all create confusion. Uncomfortable plastic chairs positively encourage "wandering". We do not have a television in the main sitting area. There is a television in a side room, which is used by those individuals who choose to watch it, usually accompanied by a member of staff. It is not a flickering screen, left on continuously, more likely to irritate than amuse.

Music is another contentious topic. We tend to rely on records and tapes rather than the radio, so that we can tailor the music to suit the activity. However, there are instances where the "chat" on the radio can be soothing to some of our centre users. As an example, we had one person with dementia who communicated regularly with the radio presenters, but who chose to ignore other service users and staff.

We have a circle of chairs around each table where tea, coffee, toast and biscuits are available on arrival at the centre, and where tea and biscuits are served before the journey home. This encourages interaction at the beginning and end of the day, and the sharing of news and gossip and reflections on the day's events. While we do invite our service users to join in, we provide alternative seating for those who do not choose to be sociable, and for those who just want a place to sit and observe the activities rather than participate themselves. Our service users no longer sit around the edge of the room with their backs to the wall – at least, not unless they choose to!

There is plenty of space provided for walking about within the centre, and we are fortunate that our centre has patio doors giving access to the gardens. We have tried to create a safe environment but must accept that persons with dementia have to be permitted to take risks. We explain to the carers, who have entrusted us with the care of their charges, that we will do our utmost to ensure that no harm befalls those who use our service, but that we cannot hope to anticipate all eventualities and at the same time allow the freedom of choice each person is entitled to.

Our staff do not wear uniforms. Some will argue that uniforms are essential to distinguish the staff from the users of the service. If our staff are indistinguishable from the users because of the lack of uniforms then we would suggest that our staff are doing an extremely good job. The persons with dementia do not have a problem with this and if another service user can meet their needs when approached, so much the better.

We have also given much attention to the activities we provide for our service users. For example, we have a "nail" box, equipped with everything required for a manicure. Some people like the staff to "do" their nails, and experience their manicure as a luxury. Others find it more satisfying to "do" their own nails, or to help another service user – so expressing their freedom and ability. Our aim is to provide but not to impose.

Baking is also a skill that we are keen for people to retain. Many of our service users have been baking all their lives and may be only too pleased to surrender the mixing bowl to someone else. We valiantly try to maintain life skills. We say: "Who would like to help us with the washing up?" While some may want to help as an expression of their capability, others may present the same response as we would receive at home – silence. Why should we expect anything different?

A learning process

We have only been able to give a brief introduction to the new culture of dementia care within our centres, and much is still to be done. It is a learning process for all of us. Training for staff working with individuals with dementia has improved enormously and attitude and approach are now seen to be as important as practical skills.

At whatever pace we choose to move forward into the new culture of dementia care, we must have regard for our staff and their needs as well as the person with dementia. We have devised a group exercise to enable staff to look at themselves as persons and respect each other's personhood. This is the starting point of our new training for those working with individuals with dementia. We all have to move forward together: persons with dementia, paid and unpaid carers and all other people who have an involvement.

We are aware that there are groups all over the country trying to work towards excellent service provision and we have, so to speak, just dipped our toes in the water. It is our strong belief that the new culture is the right way forward. To that end we will continue to involve our prime carers at every step, improving our admission procedures, breaking down barriers, recognising the person and developing appropriate care environments, with the help and support of other like-minded colleagues who share our belief in the new culture of dementia care.

References

Stone O (1992) *Awakenings*. Screenplay of Oliver Sach's book. RCA/Columbia Pictures, Los Angeles 1992.
Kitwood T (1990) The Dialectics Of Dementia: With Particular Reference to Alzheimer's Disease. *Ageing and Society* **10** 177-196.
Kitwood T & Bredin K (1992) Towards a Theory of Dementia Care. Personhood & Well Being. *Ageing and Society* **12** 269-287.

People with dementia in sheltered housing

CHAPTER
TWELVE

TRACY PETRE

Due to demographic changes and new directions in social policy, sheltered housing is set to become a major provider of accommodation for those with dementia. This chapter investigates the main problems for people with dementia and their fellow-residents in sheltered housing. It suggests ways in which sheltered housing can change so that problems can be overcome within a person-centred framework.

*T*he development of sheltered housing began in England during the post-war years as an alternative for older people to the institutions and residential homes of the early 1900s. The plan was to create grouped independent accommodation exclusively for elderly people, linked to a resident warden by an alarm system. This was a popular idea and by 1990 there were over 300,000 units of sheltered housing available in England.

The initial intention was to provide an environment for older people who were capable of living independently but were concerned about safety or sudden illness. It was emphasised that preference should be given to applicants who did not place heavy demands on wardens and other domiciliary services.

Recently though, care for elderly people has undergone great change and consequently sheltered housing will need to accommodate these changes.

New directions

The issue of sheltered housing and dementia has developed over recent years because of a combination of demographic changes and new directions in social policy. The combination of growing numbers of "old-old" during a period of reductions in provision of full-time care cannot fail to affect elderly people with extra care needs. This issue has been addressed by writers on social policy who question where people with dementia will live if their numbers are rising at a time when institutional care is declining (Keen 1992).

A key issue for providers of sheltered housing must be, whether there is any evidence to suggest that sheltered housing will become a major provider of accommodation for those with dementia. Two aspects of research would suggest this to be the case.

Recently there have been new trends in tenant populations (Carpenter *et al* 1990). Sheltered housing theoretically caters for any person over retirement age; however a study carried out recently for Anchor Housing Trust found increasingly tenants are of the old-old age group. In 1991-2, between six and 15 per cent of occupiers of sheltered housing in England were over 85 years (Rolfe et al 1993). Inevitably, if the tenant population is of this older age group the likelihood of tenants developing dementia is increased.

Secondly, qualitative data from my own research, now near completion, suggests that people with dementia may particularly gravitate to, and then stick in, this form of housing. It does not have the same provision as residential care, but even so, the tenant will not be left alone for long periods or if in great need – so it is a very attractive option for the relatives of people with mild to moderate dementia.

A popular move

Qualitative evidence suggests that family members are very eager to have a relative move into sheltered housing when there are very early signs of dementia – signs perhaps that only they can recognise. Also they generally wish for their family member to stay as long as possible when dementia develops; they may believe that this is what is best for their relative, or they may see it as a cheaper option compared to residential care. This situation means that over time increasing numbers of those with early dementia move into sheltered housing, while decreasing numbers of those with dementia move on into full time care environments.

There is reason to believe then that sheltered housing is set to become a major provider of community care for people with dementia. In order to avoid a crisis developing steps need to be taken now to ensure that life for such people occurs in line with person-centred principles. This chapter will therefore examine how dementia affects sheltered housing at present, and then will move on to discuss ways in which it can change so as to become a successful part of the new culture of dementia care.

In order for sheltered housing to become successful in terms of good community care we need to give equal consideration to the needs of three distinct groups: the tenants with dementia, the warden, and the remainder of the tenants. As each of these three groups has a major impact on the lives of the others, their problems and viewpoints need to be given equal consideration.

The needs of those with dementia

Three aspects of sheltered housing have a particular impact on the lives of those with dementia:

Lack of knowledge and understanding from others

Typically within a sheltered scheme the warden and tenants have no formal knowledge of dementia. Any knowledge base will generally be that of the myths and stereotypes propounded by the media. Scarcity of factual knowledge creates fear; for example there is a common belief that all people with dementia are aggressive, and this can lead to avoidance of the person.

A lack of knowledge also brings with it misunderstanding of so-called problem behaviours, such as wandering and aggression. Within the new culture, behaviours such as these are viewed as attempts at communication which we need to take time to read and understand. However, working alongside people with dementia in a person-centred way is not simply a matter of common sense. People need to be given insight into a person-centred approach and then given the opportunity to practise it while receiving support, encouragement and advice.

Within sheltered housing wardens rarely have had any formal training on this approach to dementia. It is even more unlikely that any of the tenants within sheltered housing would have formal knowledge on new approaches to dementia. Often, therefore, sheltered housing features a low understanding of those with dementia, combined with prejudice and alienation.

Isolation

The aim of sheltered housing is to provide, under one roof, individual self-contained units in order that tenants can decide for themselves whether they want to stay in their own flat alone, or with private visitors, or whether they want to mix with others in communal areas. Despite the fact that sheltered housing gives many opportunities for tenants to mix regularly (for example bingo and entertainment evenings) those with dementia often tend to spend the majority of their time alone in their flat.

This can be for a variety of reasons. Perhaps it is through genuine choice, based on personality: some people are not and have never been mixers, and they prefer their own company. However, there may be other reasons for a person with dementia not joining in with the group. Other tenants may no longer encourage the person with dementia to join in, or may be making them unwelcome, because they are seen as a nuisance.

For example, in my research I have encountered one scheme in which the "social core" of tenants go to the trouble to change the day and time of their domino session every week specifically so the lady with dementia in their scheme does not know when it is occurring.

Alternatively, the reasons for those with dementia not mixing may be self-initiated due to them feeling increasingly embarrassed at their inabilities, or because what is happening in the communal lounge confuses and/or frightens them. Whatever the reason people stop joining, once they do so they become isolated and have less opportunity to exercise their remaining mental powers.

Lack of orientation within the scheme

In general, sheltered housing buildings are extremely confusing. They are usually built with a number of identical floors, along which run identical doors with the flat number on each. As the communal areas are all usually on the ground floor near to the main entrance it is possible for there to be three floors and thirty identical doors between the communal lounge or main entrance and a tenants flat. During the 1980s a number of studies investigated the impact of aspects of the physical environment on those with dementia. This research particularly showed how important it was for people to find their way around if well-being was to be maintained. The sense of control over one's life is closely bound up with understanding the place one lives in (Calkins 1988).

The needs of other tenants

Thus far we have focused on the needs of those who have dementia. These are a very small minority within schemes and so now we must focus on the needs of the rest of the tenant group.

Physical safety

One of the main sources of physical danger arising from the presence of those with diminishing mental powers is that of fire. Tenants have their own cookers which could be left on, food could be forgotten while cooking, or items could fall onto hot, unattended rings. Although fire alarms and emergency procedures within sheltered housing are extremely good, all flats are joined together, with the consequence that in a serious incident fire could spread to all flats.

Other dangers relate to burglary or physical attack. It is the responsibility of each tenant within a scheme to ensure the main entrance door is locked behind them when leaving and entering, to ensure strangers are not admitted without questioning and to ensure ground floor windows are closed at night or when leaving their flat. A person who fails to do these things, possibly because of forgetting the rules, the routine, or losing a sense of the need for security, puts everyone in the building at risk.

Direct disruption from tenants with dementia

My research indicates a number of common disruptions to other tenants, for example a tenant walking into, or attempting to go into, another person's flat because they think it is their own. This usually happens because the layout of different floors is very similar.

The problem which causes the greatest amount of distress is noise at night, either because of nocturnal wandering, which other people can hear because of the building being very quiet at night, or because of the tenant ringing other people's doorbells.

A problem for certain tenants is repeated questioning or visiting for a specific reason. In many schemes one person or a small group takes on the social organising. Often the tenant with dementia will learn which person knows the day and time of any activities or trips, or to whom they should pay money for these. In these situations the tenant with dementia fixes on a question or item they need to clear up with this person and visits them repeatedly each day in an attempt to do so.

Fear of the future

Tenants who are living alongside those with dementia frequently discuss the problem that they are constantly facing the possibility that they too may develop dementia. For older people with no neurological impairment, "going senile" is probably one of their most pressing fears (Kitwood 1990). It is not surprising that tenants express the view that people with dementia should not live in the scheme.

The warden's needs

Wardens vary very much in how they perceive the problem of dementia. Three issues in particular have come to light in my research:

Lack of training and role direction

At present wardens of sheltered housing are given very little training on dementia, either during basic induction, or as more rigorous training once in post. Also they have few guidelines as to how to operate with a tenant with dementia. Therefore most wardens do not know what to expect, what will happen in the future, and how best to live alongside and support a person who does begin to show signs of dementia. Often conversation among tenants or friends leads to them acquiring negative information only, as many people have "scare stories" related to dementia which can create fear and ultimately emotional stress in wardens.

Work isolation

For many professionals working in the area of dementia care the individual carer will be working within a team of similar people, with whom they can discuss problems, let off steam, relieve tension, etc. This is very important when working in a stressful workplace. A considerable body of literature has shown that social support is related to increased psychological well-being and to a lower probability of physical illness (Cohen and Symes 1985).

In comparison to this the majority of wardens of sheltered schemes work alone, and it is their lone responsibility to deal with tenants with dementia. This situation could lead to wardens beginning to develop the emotional problems and psychological ill-being which have been well researched and catalogued as occurring in family carers of those with dementia, who are similarly at risk of becoming isolated.

Lack of role awareness from others

A large problem which faces wardens is that other professional groups, which hold power and service allocation, for example GPs and social services departments, often do not have clear knowledge of the warden's role.

This leads to situations in which tenants are discharged from hospital when not fully recovered and capable of independent living, because it is assumed the warden's role is to look after his or her tenants, and to oversee medication, etc. Similarly services can be withheld from those in sheltered housing because it is often assumed that tenants can manage without the full neccessary care package, since the warden will do extra tasks for the person.

Where these wrong assumptions by other professional groups exist, wardens increasingly become misused and have unnecessary burdens placed upon them. This applies especially to situations where tenants are mentally frail and in need of extra support.

Moving forward

These problems cannot be removed overnight. Nevertheless preliminary findings from my research suggest that sheltered housing can provide a very successful environment for maintaining the well-being and personhood of tenants with dementia; and more importantly, that this is not linked to the severity of the condition measured in cognitive terms.

The key factor is the quality of the social milieu in a particular sheltered scheme, and this relates primarily to the attitudes and feelings of the warden and other tenants. Certain relatively small changes could be implemented to remove many of the problems and create a more person-centred environment for tenants with dementia. Some of these changes refer mainly to the organisation, and some more to the promotion of good care within an individual scheme.

Changes for the organisation

The evidence I have brought forward suggests that the warden's role needs to be much more clearly defined if dementia care becomes a part of the work. This will help the warden feel supported and may also help them avoid becoming involved in extra help-giving for certain tenants, which then becomes difficult to stop. Ultimately this will lead to less emotional strain on wardens who know they are fully supported by their housing association/authority when they have to say, "No I can't do that."

Informing other professionals

It is also necessary for the warden's role to be more strongly promoted. All providers of sheltered housing need to make a large and vociferous effort to inform GPs, hospital staff, social services, voluntary organisations and family members, of exactly what the role of a warden is, and what he or she can and can't be expected to do for mentally frail tenants. Only when this information becomes common knowledge will service providers stop making assumptions about what the warden is supposed to do and will begin both to put in the full range of services the person with dementia is entitled to, and to co-operate and communicate with the warden as a fellow professional.

Training

Wardens need specialist training related to dementia, if the new culture of dementia care is to extend into sheltered housing. Some factual information is needed, but above all else they need to know how to relate to those who have dementia as persons with particular abilities and vulnerabilities. If wardens have this insight and knowledge the message can be filtered through to other tenants, making it possible for a person-centred environment to develop.

Wardens need much stronger social support if they are to be expected to be involved with providing accommodation for those with dementia. This includes bringing wardens in local areas together to talk, share problems and advise; in other words to fulfill the role which other support groups have in reducing emotional stress and psychological ill-health.

Changes at an individual scheme level

Providers who design and build sheltered housing which caters for those with dementia need to be aware of the important benefits of clarity and ease of orientation on this group. Very minor adaptations such as colour coding and sign posting will have an effect on the ability of those with dementia to find their way around, and will decrease the likelihood of them mistaking other people's flats for their own. This will have important knock-on effects in increasing everyone's well-being.

As discussed earlier it is important to recognise that tenants with dementia may become isolated against their wishes. It would generally be agreed within the new culture of dementia care that people with dementia can receive a lot of benefit from spending time with others who are sensitive to their needs and abilities. Sheltered housing has two important resources for creating an active social environment for those with dementia: a communal lounge, together with large numbers of other tenants who in the majority have a lot of spare time. Wardens need to be trained to utilise these resources to the best effect, to encourage willing and able tenants to chat with those with dementia, to join in activities with them, to pop in and visit them and to invite them to activities.

Finally, voluntary organisations such as the Alzheimer's Disease Society can be a very useful link for wardens, depending on the strength of the group in the individual area. They can provide emotional support, information, and, a practical knowledge base for the warden, and may also be able to visit the scheme to run activities, day care, etc, which tenants could join.

Sheltered housing in the new culture

The preliminary findings of my research suggest that the physical environment a person with dementia lives in is less important than the social environment. Those with dementia need positive human contact from people who value their individuality, needs, and desires. Sheltered housing can change to fit into this role provided there are:

• training for the warden on a person-centred approach to dementia
• strong links with support and service providers
• clarity and ease of orientation in the physical design of the building.

On taking this point of view I do not wish to suggest that sheltered housing is, or could become, the ideal environment for people with dementia to live in. We simply need to face reality, and tackle the problems while they remain small and manageable. The roots of a new culture of dementia care within sheltered housing need to be laid now.

References

Keen J (1992) *Dementia*. Office of Health Economics
Carpenter I *et al* (1990) *Housing Care and Frailty*. Anchor Housing Trust, Oxford.
Rolfe S, Mackintosh S, Leather P (1993) *Age File '93*. Anchor Housing Trust, Oxford.
Calkins M (1988) *Design for Dementia: Planning Environments for the Elderly and the Confused*. National Health Publishing, Owings Mills, Maryland.
Kitwood T (1990) The Dialectics of Dementia: With Particular Reference to Alzheimer's Disease. *Ageing and Society* **10** 177-196.
Cohen S, Syme SL (1985) *Social Support and Health*. Harcourt Brace Jovanovich, London & New York..

CHAPTER THIRTEEN | Involving volunteers in care provision

ROSAS MITCHELL

Two very different, innovative schemes provided by volunteers are described here. One is a town centre drop-in cafe for people who are in the early stages of dementia and their carers. The other is a day out to the home of a volunteer as part of a small group of people who have dementia. The paper looks at the unique contribution volunteers can bring to dementia care and considers some of the principles involved.

Recent changes in organisation of health and social services have given us the opportunity to develop small and innovatory services to meet the individual needs of people with dementia and their carers. An increasing role is to be provided by the voluntary sector who have a long tradition in providing cost effective services which are well suited to users' needs. Voluntary sector projects have also been able to attract additional resources such as central government grants.

In Central Region, Scotland, which has a population of 272,000 covering three main urban centres and a vast rural area, it was decided to set up a post to develop a wide range of services for people with dementia and their carers. This was my particular challenge in the Autumn of 1991. I was an employee of the local authority, working in partnership with health board, social work and the voluntary sector and the post was funded through the specific mental illness grant.

In recognition of the wide diversity of individual need, it was hoped to provide a broad range of services. Some have looked at developing existing services. This was the case of a local residential home which set up flexible day and evening care, flexible respite breaks and more recently long-term specialist care, thus providing a continuum of care within the one resource.

The Mobile Emergency Care Scheme is another example. This has a long tradition of providing help through mobile wardens to isolated people within their own homes. However, the service assumes that people can call for help when it is needed, so it was often not appropriate for people with dementia. A new scheme was set up which provides passive alarms within the home. This means help can be immediately available if people are wandering at night or there is a fire, gas leak or the possibility of hypothermia.

Other projects have been piloted in which people become self-employed and commit themselves to providing flexible respite care either in their own home or the home of the person with dementia. A further extension of this is the provision of long term care in the community in which paid carers take people into their homes and care for them on a one-to-one basis in a domestic setting. These homes are registered for residential care and are paid at the DSS rates for residential care.

The wide range of services developed has contributed towards filling some of the gaps and helped to give people increased choice. Some of the most successful have been run by volunteers and it is these services which I want to describe in more detail.

Drop-In Cafe

The "Town Break" Drop-In Cafe was the vision of a group of carers and former carers in the Stirling area. It was to provide a resource for people in the early stages of dementia and support for their relatives. They recognised this gap in the services and tackled it by coming together with a group of people from a town centre church who made their ground floor facilities available for one day a week.

A partnership developed between the Church and the Alzheimer Scotland Action on Dementia Support Group, their development worker and the Dementia Initiative Worker. As a result a relaxed cafe environment was created which is acceptable to both carers and people with dementia. Carers can find information, support and counselling, as well as friendship with other carers. When happy to leave their relative, they can take the opportunity to shop or have a break in town: thus it provides a respite service.

For the person with dementia, it is probably the first experience of services. However, the informality, the absence of records and assessments and the opportunity to come along when you feel like it are very acceptable. There are a wide range of appropriate activities but many enjoy the opportunity to chat on a one to one basis with a volunteer. This is an opportunity to share and to feel you are really listened to and accepted. Many find it very difficult to come to terms with what is happening to them and recognise they are with people who understand.

Town Break, like many new services, had a very slow start. It takes a long time to establish credibility, especially when the model of care is very new.

However, after two and a half years, it is a thriving resource with an average of ten people with dementia coming along each week. Many come with their carers, others come with a volunteer or make their own way to the cafe. There are usually about seven or eight carers popping in during the day. Some who are working in the town, take the opportunity to join their relative for the simple snack lunch that is provided.

As the resource has grown, other services have developed to meet need. For example, it was recognised that there were a few carers who would like more in-depth support and counselling. A group was established each week led by a retired psychologist from the local carer's forum which could help carers look at the emotional needs of caring. Some weeks the group is for those currently caring and other weeks it aims to support those who have released their relative to hospital or residential long term care. Carers who use the resource have also enjoyed the opportunity to take part in carers' education days. This has been acceptable because they knew and trusted the people organising it.

Another service which has evolved from the Drop-In Cafe is a befriending service for people with dementia. This happened very naturally as volunteers became aware of the isolation and loneliness of some of the people who attended the resource and extended their friendship to them at other times. This service was formalised during the last few months and a co-ordinator appointed who could recruit, train and support volunteers. The scheme is available in the rural areas of Stirling District where people currently have little in the way of support.

The Town Break "drop-in" model has been successfully adopted in other town centres in the Region. Each one has developed its own structure and identity to meet local need. In all cases, co-ordinators are appointed to be responsible for the overall running of the day and the selection, training and support of the volunteers. Funding, in all cases, has come through the Specific Mental Illness Grant.

Home from home

"Home from home" is another service which has developed with a strong contribution from volunteers. Volunteers open their homes and, supported by a relative or friend, they offer a day out once or twice a week to up to four or five people, all of whom have some degree of dementia. It was a response to the need for some specialist day care in one of the urban areas of Central Region and was the result of a lengthy consultation process with people with dementia, carers and professionals from a wide variety of backgrounds.

The model that emerged was the one that was felt to offer the best opportunity for people with dementia to feel accepted, integrated and normal. It was called "home day care" but this proved to be a misleading name. It is more about a special day out to a friend's house.

"Home from home" is a very exciting scheme which has now been operational for two and a half years and has spread to many areas of the Region. One of the important features which makes it successful for people with dementia is its size. Each group has four or five members. This means that each member has the opportunity to find someone there that they can really relate to but doesn't feel overwhelmed by the large numbers. Each group has two or three home day carers thus offering a good ratio of care and the opportunity to relate and work on a one to one basis.

People are very much seen as individuals with their own needs and rights. Outings and excursions are much easier to arrange for a small number and can take place on the spur of the moment. The small numbers make this model of day care very appropriate for rural areas and also for targeting different age groups. All the group members come from the same surrounding locality which helps to provide a rich resource of material for reminiscence and discussion. It also prevents people having to spend a long time travelling. Transport is provided by volunteer drivers in their own cars and this helps to give the person collected a sense of normality as the "welfare bus" is not used.

It is this normality which people with dementia crave for. The opportunity to continue in their own homes with their own routines and to feel that they still have a purpose in their lives. Going out for the day with friends is an experience most of us have enjoyed all our lives and "Home from home" gives an opportunity for it to continue. The normal, homely environment with the comfortable chairs, coal fires, family atmosphere with pre-school children involved or school children coming home at lunch time, family pets of all descriptions, all help to give a relaxed atmosphere in which people can be themselves and feel valued and important. Small children with their ability to be non-judgemental, open and affectionate, have been a very important part of "Home from home".

The home environment is so important. There is so much stimulation at hand which can never be found in the normal residential or community day care settings. Home day carers feel very relaxed in their own homes with everything they need in easy reach. Activities can be the very normal things one does in one's own home – preparing meals, setting tables, washing up, gardening, looking at photos, going for walks. In this way, the activities of daily living can be maintained, skills sustained and abilities and hobbies encouraged.

Right from the start people need to make the choice about attending the group. Introductions are done gradually and take time so the person feels comfortable with the concept. Personal histories are requested from the carers so that the home day carers have the opportunity to know as much as possible about the person's biography and particularly how they have coped with loss in their lives. Once at the group, they are treated as individuals who are given independence and choices. The tremendous amount of acceptance and respect given to group members makes them feel valued and affirmed.

At the end of the day, most of the group members have forgotten all the details. The important issues surround whether they go home with a sense of self worth and feelings of contentment. Have their experiences made them feel they counted as people and their opinion mattered? Were they made to feel they could actually make things happen and ultimately, did they have a feeling of "trust" because of where they had been and who they had been with? These four criteria outlined by Kitwood and Bredin (1992) are important questions when attempting to evaluate a service.

Carers are invited from the outset to be part of the partnership of "Home from home". They are invited to visit with their relative and drop in at any time. Home day carers develop close relationships with some carers. Other carers prefer to be less involved but always with the knowledge that they can approach the project worker or home day carer with any concern and that they have access to a complaints procedure.

Using volunteers

This is not the place to discuss the reasons for the government's policy of extending the role of the voluntary sector. It is the culture in which we work, and we must maximise the benefits it can bring for the person with dementia. It is certainly true that we are able to do a lot more because we are working with volunteers, and can therefore provide cost effective services. At the same time we should not minimise the quality and suitability of their contribution.

Volunteers, on the whole, are ordinary, normal people. People with dementia desperately want to be treated as ordinary, normal people and volunteers are free to do just that. Home day carers all insist that they see their group members as individual friends who are treated as equals and this is very evident to see.

The closeness of the group often gives the person with dementia the opportunity to be the one who offers support, who gives comfort or who assists others. Often, a group member sees him or herself as the helper in the group. Volunteers are not affected by status or boundaries, professional allegiance or objectivity. They can become real friends, accepting people as they are and offering their own vulnerability and weakness.

Volunteers choose to work in this area. They want to work with people with dementia. Nobody twisted their arm or forced them. They come of their own volition, each one motivated by a variety of different reasons.

However, the new culture of dementia care has given us hope, quality and the opportunity to see improvement. It is now a very positive field to be committed to, knowing that your input is vital and the rewards, though sometimes small, are definitely there. The challenge to be creative, the give and take of relationships and the opportunity to participate in a group all help to provide motivation. One home day carer recently commented on her commitment "I do it for the sheer pleasure of it".

One of the serious reservations concerning "Home from Home" was whether you could provide a reliable service using volunteers. Our experience has been that people's commitment is overwhelming. They have really grasped the need for continuity, reliability and commitment. People have left their friends to continue using their homes while they are away on holiday or they have helped each other out so that people will not be without a service. This experience has been confirmed by Anne Connor's study of community care projects run by voluntary sector agencies (Connor 1994).

There can be no doubt that the more carer time we can achieve for each individual with dementia, the better the opportunity for a quality service. The use of volunteers within services means that we are able to offer more individualised care, more diversity with the range of skills that can be offered, more time to listen and moretime to do quality things together. Much of the success of the drop-in cafe is due to the fact that the number of volunteers always allows people to have someone they can sit down and talk to on their own.

Despite gloomy forecasts about the dwindling pool of volunteers, there has never been a problem with recruitment for either "Town Break" or "Home from home". Many of the volunteers are in their fifties or sixties, either early retired or newly retired, who are looking to make a contribution to the community. Mothers who are staying at home to bring up a family or those working part time are another valuable group. Our policy is not to take on people who are actively looking for work, as we are hoping for a reasonable length of commitment.

The majority of volunteers come with some experience of caring and many have been former carers. They have often acquired a wealth of knowledge and expertise which they are anxious to put to further use. They have a lot to teach professionals and their sharing may help them to make some sense of their own personal tragedy.

Vital principles
In running services for volunteers, a few important principles need to be adhered to. Firstly, there is **ownership**. Ideally, it is good if the volunteers can be

there from the beginning. This was the case with the "Town Break" cafe. The majority of the volunteers who helped create and structure the resource, are still there working in it two and a half years later. They remember the bewilderment, isolation and confusion when their relative was in the initial stages of the illness. They now want to provide for current carers a resource which they would have longed to have. The resource belongs to the volunteers.

In the "Home from home" project, the volunteers also have a very strong sense of ownership. This is because it is held in their own home and they have equal status with their friend or relative with whom they are working. Together, they create the atmosphere, decide on activities and determine how the day will be structured. Although support and advice is available, it is very much the volunteers' day and the creativity and responsibility rests with them. A resource library of books, training packs, games, tapes and videos is available to the volunteers to use in their own homes.

Secondly, **training** must be an essential ingredient if volunteers are going to feel confident with their new responsibilities. A training package is offered before people are accepted as volunteers and a three day course covers various aspects of dementia care. It is a valuable time to look at attitudes and abilities and to assess gaps in knowledge and the need for further training. People have the opportunity to withdraw if they feel it is not for them and counselling can be offered at this point. Once people are accepted onto the projects, training and support continue. There are regular meetings, some of which are support and sharing, some more formal training and some provide reviews. It is important that at all times the volunteer feels supported and can find advice and information readily.

Volunteers also need individual **support** to cope with the stresses of the illness and should always be given the opportunity to withdraw before burn-out or exhaustion set in.

Good support and training give the volunteer a sense of self worth and value and an affirmation of the importance of what they are doing. This is extremely important in the absence of monetary reward, and can happen in many and varied ways. Good working relationships with professionals working in the field of dementia help to raise the profile of the schemes. In both the "Town Break" and "Home from home" there was continuous involvement from the planning stage through to training and then continuous visits and support once the project was up and running. Constant referrals from these professionals give volunteers a sense of the value of their scheme and their partnership with professionals.

It is important that volunteers feel they are part of something which is dynamic, vibrant and meeting need. The "Town Break" drop-in cafe has twenty volunteers.

People enjoy being there, and that is crucial.

There are many other practical ways of affirming the value of volunteers. These include things like offering expenses and making sure they are paid promptly and willingly. In "Home from Home", volunteers are paid according to the number of people attending and they can receive up to £49 for the day. This helps to cover extra heating, food, drink, equipment, wear and tear, travel expenses etc. Volunteers need to know that they are insured for all eventualities and that aids and adaptations are available if needed.

A good selection process also helps to show that you value your volunteers as well as set high standards for your schemes. Applicants to "Home from home" are assessed over a period of time and references and medical opinion as to suitability are sought. The home is assessed by an occupational therapist, and fire precaution measures are installed. A final visit is made with a local social worker and a report submitted to a panel made up of a principal professional officer (day care and residential care) a community psychiatric nurse, a carer, a representative from a voluntary organisation and a social worker. If accepted, the volunteers are provided with a letter of appointment, a service description and comprehensive guidelines.

Evaluation, monitoring, regular reviews of schemes and continual review of placements in "Home from home" help affirm to the volunteers the importance of their work and show where it fits in with the greater scheme of helping people with dementia and their carers.

Conclusion

These schemes came out of a small amount of money for development and a blank piece of paper. They started with the person with dementia themselves and not the existing services. They are based on principles of trust, openness, user involvement and normal living experiences.

The services hope to be liberating and creative rather than controlling, and aim to involve people as whole people valued and accepted as equals. The person-centred approach has helped to make them into quality services and this has an impact on people's ability to cope. If we provide "good" services then people do better. These schemes show us that this can be especially true when the care in the community is care by the community.

References

Kitwood T and Bredin K (1992) Towards a Theory of Dementia Care: Personhood and Well-being. *Ageing and Society* 12 269-287.
Connor A (1994) "The Role of the Voluntary Sector in the New Community Care Arrangements". In Titterton M (Ed) *Caring for People in the Community*. Jessica Kingsley, London. p143.

CHAPTER FOURTEEN

A new pattern of life: re-assessing the role of occupation and activities

TESSA PERRIN

The role and value of occupation in the health care of persons with severe dementia is briefly appraised. The author calls for the establishing of an occupational model to inform and structure the treatment of dementia, and suggests occupations whose therapeutic potential requires investigation.

*I*t always seemed to me that Grace was so fragile she would break if she was moved. She never did of course; but I think other staff felt the same, for she was always handled like fine porcelain. She was thin, skeletal almost, and her skin had that bluish translucency through which the blood vessels stand out clearly. She lay all day on a recliner chair with a sheepskin beneath her, feet wrapped up in thick woolly bedsocks. To my knowledge she had neither language nor verbalisation of any kind. She was blind, and she rarely initiated movement, purposeful or otherwise. She appeared to have reached that stage of dementia which has been termed the vegetative state.

Grace was in a small unit for those with very severe dementia. My brief was to work with staff on the unit, trying to address the poverty of environmental stimulation. Grace responded to nothing, until one day I place a large rag doll against her as she lay in her chair, nestling its head into her neck. Almost as a natural reflex, Grace's arms slowly went about the doll, holding it to her breast. As we watched, the fingers of one hand went into the stranded woollen hair, winding and tangling it around. The other hand went to the dress, smoothing and patting and rearranging the folds. When lunchtime came, she wouldn't let it go.

By contrast, May was a soul in whom the fire was still very much alive; a damaged lady to be sure, but still possessed of a vitality, a spark that could and would ignite on provocation. May had no language of any real utility, except for a few pungent obscenities when the mood was upon her. But verbalise she did, invariably at times of anger or distress. She would shout and yell until somebody attended her, at which point she would launch into an excited explanation of what was troubling her, which went something like this: "I said sai sai ssa ssa sss sss, and she she sh sh sh. And I ffa ffa ff ff ff". Beyond I said and he/she said, language evaded her. These communications were attended sometimes by tears, sometimes by a shaken fist, and she was not averse to giving a clump on the ear or a bite on the arm

to anyone attempting to handle her at such a time.

At all other times of the waking day, May would sit quite still and passive. She would engage in no constructive activity of any kind other than sometimes feeding herself, but she remained alert, and engaged eye contact easily. I and my care staff colleagues had tried all kinds of approaches to divert May from her rages, and indeed from her passivity. She was either at one extreme or the other, neither of which seemed to hold any positive experience for her. Music, singing, art, crafts, video; all these left her cold. Then one day I took a ball into the room and started to throw and bounce it around. Immediately she came alive, laughing and hurling it at me with great glee.

Encouraged by such a vital response, I took a tin of bubble mixture in with me the next day. She looked starstruck as the room filled with bubbles, then surprised as they burst cold against her skin. She seemed affronted as I blew bubbles at her, and started to blow back; we had a bubble fight and she began to laugh and bat them about and clap them between her hands. Her legs waggled about in front of her as she jiggled up and down in her chair. She was totally involved in a bubble experience. From where I sat, it looked extraordinarily close to something that might just be called joy.

Childish and undignified?

Dolls? Ball games? Bubbles? Ten, or perhaps even five years ago I would not have countenanced the use of such activities in my work as occupational therapist to elderly people in long-term care. I considered them demeaning and insulting, simplistic, childish and undignified. They neither stretch nor challenge the client. They ignore the holistic stance so beloved of occupational therapy. They have no concern with functional independence. They have nothing to do with rehabilitation. Last but perhaps not least, I was embarrassed to use them in front of my colleagues.

Such were the old attitudes, the traditional reasoning, stemming from a training now some 20 years in the past, and a long experience of the mental health field in which maturity, responsibility, independence and self-control were the pre-eminent goals of therapy. And then eight years ago I found myself, more by circumstance than design, pitched into the deep end of dementia care and floundering. My brief was to provide a service to 13 residential homes for elderly people; large, institutional, 60-bedded homes. I had no helpers, no equipment, no resources, no budget. In fact, I was a mug to take the task on board.

But how very glad I am that I did, for though I could have no realisation of it then, it was the beginning of what has been the most exciting and rewarding, painful and frustrating journey of my life. There have been challenges at every corner: to the efficacy of my therapeutic practice, to my credibility as practitioner, and indeed to the very adequacy of my own personhood. But what this has led me to has been a reappraisal of the role of occupational therapy in dementia care, to a new and altered stance of therapeutic practice, and to the pursuit of those occupational approaches which elicit and sustain well-being in elderly people with dementia. In short, I have had (and am having) to rethink my chosen profession, at least in so far as it impinges upon dementia care.

A new pattern of therapy

As I assumed this new role, it became clear that other members of the multi-disciplinary team were looking to me to produce and implement therapies that would "work". There was an expectation that while others might "care", I must "make better". The past eight years have been a search to discover those treatments that do make better; a fundamental question behind the search being, "What do we mean by make better?"

With the less seriously impaired older person who is living at home or who is returning home from short-term care, the standard theoretical approaches and practices remain appropriate: we are concerned with every facet of the client's being, and we are encouraging their return to an optimum independence of function.

But for the person in long-term care, our emphasis must necessarily be different. For myself, the issue is no longer "how to increase independence" or "how to restore function", but "how to make happy". My concern is now more to do with the client's being, rather than doing. The losses experienced by the person in an advanced dementia are so devastating and all-pervasive, that ability (or lack of it) becomes somehow irrelevant. What is surely of overwhelming importance is comfort, contentment, well-being. Making better is still the central objective, but it is making feel better, rather than making do better.

A new pattern of assessment

If the focus of therapy has changed, the style of assessment must adjust accordingly. Traditionally, the occupational therapist will attempt a comprehensive assessment of need, generally framed in terms of that which a client can or cannot do. What self-care tasks has this mentally handicapped woman not yet learned? How can this person with a stroke adapt his leisure pursuits to accommodate his disability? What work roles and skills have been affected by this man's depressive illness? And in order to facilitate the assessment, most therapists have to hand a range of assessment tests, schedules and batteries, both standardised and "home-made".

For the person with severe dementia this approach is redundant. Of course, we do need to have an overall awareness of level of function, in order that we may approach sensitively, and encourage toward success rather than failure in those tasks which can still be attempted. But if the prime objective of our intervention is *feeling* better, we need some kind of measure of being rather than of doing, of emotion rather than action. How can such an entity be measured? Who can know what another is feeling? We really have only one avenue open to us.

Unlike the doctor who investigates both signs (external evidences of ill health) and symptoms (sensations experienced by the patient), we are usually unable to ascertain symptoms. We are dealing predominantly with psychological state, and most of our clients are unable to articulate abstract concepts such as emotion. So we are dependent upon signs, those outward manifestations of inner state. Until comparatively recently, our observations of those signs have necessarily been somewhat subjective. However, the recent advent of dementia care mapping (see chapter 15) has offered a well-validated, structured assessment which enables us to build some objectivity into our assessment. It not only indicates the signs we should be looking for, it also gives the person with dementia something of a voice with which his symptoms may be articulated. It helps us to know how a person feels now; and when we have applied our intervention, it helps us to detect if he feels better.

A new pattern of training

There is within most long-stay settings some understanding that activities are "A Good Thing". Whenever I request clarification of this view in practice or in training, common responses are "It gives them something to do with their hands" or "It keeps their minds occupied" or "They need to keep busy" (interesting that activities are for "them", not for us). On such an impoverished theory base are most activity programmes built.

It is probably true to say that most activities run in long-stay settings are carried out by unqualified staff, only some of whom are trained in good care practice, and very few of whom have been trained in the appropriate use of occupation. It perhaps says something about the priority given by training departments to the role and value of occupation in health care. And maybe too, it says something even more significant about occupational therapy as a profession; that it has not yet effectively declared what it has to offer dementia care.

My own belief is that occupation (purposeful activity) is a fundamental human need, critical to health and wholeness. Impose constraints upon a person's daily occupations, through ill health, disability, redundancy, imprisonment... and the negative effects on physical and psychological well-being are very soon apparent. Conversely, the application of appropriate occupation in situations of occupational deprivation or dysfunction acts as a natural restorative to function and well-being (Kielhofner 1985).

Over the last 10-15 years, an expanded body of theory supporting these contentions has developed, culminating in the recent emergence of occupational science (Yerxa 1993) as a new discipline having the potential to articulate the role and value of occupation in health care as never before. Its place in other disciplines, such as physical disability, mental handicap and mental health, is well known. The time is surely ripe therefore for occupational therapy to stand up and be counted as a valued instrument in the treatment of disability and ill-being in dementia. It is no longer good enough to charge unqualified, untrained staff with the task of applying occupations to dementia care. We would not expect such staff to prescribe or administer drugs. The misapplication of occupations can damage people just as surely as the misapplication of drugs.

This is a priority area of need in training. Staff must understand and appreciate the role and value of occupation in health and dementia care. They must know how to apply occupation to individual and group need. They must be able to administer occupation sensitively and effectively. They must be able to evaluate the therapeutic process. To be sure, they do not have to become occupational therapists; but they must become competent practitioners of applied occupation in dementia care. It is my firm belief that if as much training time were allocated to occupational care as it is to physical care, we would be seeing considerably less ill-being, and managing considerably fewer behavioural problems in those of our clients advanced in dementia.

A new pattern of occupations

As in every other facet of being, the person with dementia is occupationally impaired. The dementia may initially manifest itself in a reduced work efficiency, particularly where the work has a significant cognitive component. It advances insidiously, affecting hobbies and leisure interests, which will in time be put aside in frustration, disinterest or despair. Latterly, even ingrained life-long self-care routines suffer, and it might be true to say that the person's very occupational nature has changed. Occupations which once held meaning and purpose, no longer do so.

The challenge for us, as for the person with dementia, is one of adaptation. We seek not to return him to what he was, but to help him adapt to what he is. The young man with a severe spinal cord lesion may initially hope to walk again and to resume his previous occupations. To be thinking this way after two years would indicate a maladaptive response. Health and well-being lie in acceptance of the disability and adaptation to it, on the part of his carers as well as himself. It is no different for the dementia sufferer and his carers.

Restoring a person to past skills and abilities may have some relevance in the early stages of dementia, where insight is retained and disability minimal, but it is not appropriate in advanced dementia. We need to recognise that much of what we have offered in the past by way of therapeutic intervention is not only not helpful, it may be quite damaging.

First, we need to reconsider our use of those cognitive approaches which are so commonly used in elderly care, for example reality orientation, reminiscence, quizzes, discussion. All may be effective therapeutic approaches, but very demanding of memory and intellectual function. The stress that they can exert upon the person whose intellectual faculties are now diminished and disordered, is not inconsiderable. We should have particular concern about the use of reality orientation; an effective therapy with certain individuals in certain circumstances, but for the person who has retreated to a different, more comfortable reality than the one in which you and I live, it can be counter-productive, distressing and damaging. My personal view is that we must reject these cognitive approaches in severe dementia.

Second, we must think through our use of craft based occupations. The value of craft activities lies in a tangible, well-crafted end product. However, the person in advanced dementia is generally much reduced in practical ability and manual dexterity. You and I might not mind if our client drops stitches, splodges paint and dribbles on pristine fabric, but are we quite sure they don't? Long-term memory is quite a long time departing; a poorly-worked end product, once fashioned with skill and ease, but now requiring maximum supervision throughout the process, is only reinforcing declining ability and draining self-esteem.

So in effect, this knocks out a large portion of those occupations commonly available. What is left to us? What we need to do is to look at occupations which are not skill based, nor dependent on quality output. We need to bear in mind that dementia seems to attack output mechanisms (skills, performance, action) and the intellectual processes which underpin them. It seems to leave intact primary input mechanisms (the six senses) and the emotions which can appreciate them. Dementia care needs to give more attention, I believe, to sensory deprivation theory.

Bower (1967) and Bexton (1954) demonstrated radical effects of sensory deprivation upon the physical and psychological well-being of volunteers; confusion and disorientation being the prominent features. Implicit in their studies was the hypothesis that if a sensorily deprived environment can induce confusion and disorientation, sensorily enhanced environments should reduce or at least restrain the advance of confusion and disorientation.

I believe this is an area of dementia care research long overdue. The recent interest in the use of multisensory equipment with elderly people is a step in the right direction, but it is an expensive therapy, and needs looking at carefully. Some research has been done (Moffat *et al* 1993) but there are many other questions requiring answers. It is clear though, that this needs to be the nub of future research: what occupations are most effective in using a person's sensory avenues to induce well-being?

I think we need to look at the place of music and dance, physical exercise and physical games. We must investigate tactile approaches such as massage, facials and manicure, and perhaps the handling of pets. Aromatherapy would appear to have therapeutic potential. We should consider too, those multi-sensory occupations such as cooking, gardening, flower arranging, which although task and skill based may perhaps also be adapted, and utilised from a predominantly sensory point of view. In my own practice, I use and have observed many of these approaches, and know in my heart that they have a real utility in dementia care. I have seen them "work". I can relate anecdotes in demonstration. I am sure many other practitioners can do likewise. However, they remain as yet unproven. We have not tested, not investigated, not researched. We actually know very little about the therapeutic potential and worth of these approaches. This is a task which we must address with some urgency.

A new pattern of life

It cannot be denied that until very recently, "life" for most elderly people in long-stay care, has consisted in daily 12 hour periods of chair-sitting (or possibly corridor-pacing), punctuated spasmodically by brief food or toilet experiences. It cannot be denied that there are yet many, many long-stay settings where that is still the sum total of "life" for residents. For you and me it would be unthinkable to sit for one day staring at the wall, let alone days that turn into months and years. Yet this is still the generally accepted norm for our parents and grandparents in long-term care. It is a situation so common that few challenge it.

But thankfully, the tide is turning. We have faced the very complex problems of advanced dementia and tried all sorts of ways to deal with them. We have ignored them and hoped they would go away, but they don't. We have chastised and felt ashamed. We have used tranquillising drugs and know that these are rarely the answer. We have used restraint or isolation, but we know that this solves nothing. We have tried RO and found it doesn't work (Stokes & Goudie 1990).

Increasingly though, there are practitioners who are challenging previous norms, who are learning how to care for people with dementia, and who are working to share new knowledge and fresh insights (Kitwood & Bredin 1992). We have thought a little more about the true nature of confusion and dementia. We have understood a little more about the malign processes of institutionalisation. We have discovered a little more about ourselves and the way people interact with us. We have used the tools we have, and found them wanting. And thus we edge towards an understanding of what effective dementia care is all about.

I believe that there is however, a major step ahead of us; and that is that we need with some urgency an evaluation of an occupational model for use in dementia care. The nursing model is inadequate; physical care is only one part of a very large whole. The medical model is inappropriate; our clients are not sick, nor are they necessarily "terminal". They are disabled. Most of them are living in seriously impoverished environments. If is is possible to starve to death psychologically, that is exactly what is happening.

For myself, life and health consists in work that gives me a sense of purpose, in hobbies that enable me to create, in leisure interests that bring me pleasure and fun, and in relationships in which I find warmth, love and security. I am sure it is the same for you. Should it not be the same for the person with dementia?

When we have learned how to discover or adapt those occupations which will offer the older person those same qualities of life that we all expect and consider our right, we will I believe, have found the key to sustained well-being in dementia. In practice, it means that we are going to have to learn how to fill satisfactorily those hours spent staring at the wall, and there are many of them. We are going to have to transform the client's occupational day. It is major task. But perhaps we might sustain ourselves in that task by knowing that while the medics might be adding years to life, we are adding life to years.

References

Bexton WH, Heron W, Scott TH (1954) Effects of decreased variation in the sensory environment. *Canadian Journal of Psychology* **8 (2)** 70-76.

Bower HM (1967) Sensory stimulation and the treatment of senile dementia. *Medical Journal of Australia* **1(22)** 1113-1119.

Kielhofner G (1983) *Health through occupation: theory and practice in occupational therapy.* FA Davis, Philadelphia.

Kitwood T, Bredin K (1992) *Person to Person.* Gale Centre Publications.

Moffat N, Barker P, Pinkney L, Garside M, Freeman C (1993) *Snoezelen: an Experience for People with Dementia.* Dorset Healthcare NHS Trust.

Stokes G, Goudie F (1990) *Working with Dementia.* Winslow Press, Bicester.

Yerxa EJ (1993) Occupational science: a new source of power for participants in occupational therapy. *Occupational Science: Australia,* **April 1(1)** 3-10.

Mapping the advance of the new culture in dementia care

LINDA FOX

The method and practice of dementia care mapping are explained in detail. The results of two comprehensive studies in day care centres are discussed and contrasted to emphasise the extent of the new culture in dementia care.

*I*f it is really the case that a new culture in dementia care is emerging, we need means to identify how far this has come about. Dementia care mapping (known as DCM) is one such method. In this chapter, I will discuss some of the findings from two of Bradford Dementia Group's most recent and comprehensive evaluations of day care, using the DCM method. The main issues relating to care practice arising from the evaluations will be discussed, together with matters relating to staff support. Finally, I will comment on the experience of evaluating.

At present, the dementia care environment is in a continual state of flux as a result of changes in policy, management structure, staffing, resource levels, etc. Despite much that works against improvement, it is remarkable that many changes are occurring so as to meet the real needs of persons with dementia – this is a small step towards better quality care. These are but the beginnings; there is a long way yet to go before a new culture is established.

The DCM method

DCM is an observational method used to evaluate the quality of care in formal settings. To observe care environments with as little disruption as possible, and after informal introductions, mappers need to merge gently into the setting by situating themselves alongside the persons with dementia. To gain the best results from mapping data, observation, and in some cases involvement (especially in the case of tea break and mealtimes) are necessary, on an equal human level. Privacy, however, needs to be respected at all times.

Interaction can take place between mappers, clients and staff throughout the evaluation. It is crucial to reassure, provide answers to questions, or clarify any points that clients or staff may request, in an open and honest way. If a person with dementia asks the reason for a mapper's presence, for example, then it would be appropriate to say something like "we are here to find out how it is for you and see if any improvements can be made". Any interaction between client and mapper is noted in the data collected.

A short de-briefing with staff at the end of each day can also help to clear up any concerns or queries and alleviate any apprehension. Higher quality data can be gained by mapping as much of the day, over as many days, as is possible.

The principle underlying DCM is that the observer should at all times take the standpoint of the person with dementia to gain an empathic sense of what his or her life may be like. As one of the founder-users of the method, Elizabeth Barnett, has put it: "To learn the DCM method is to acquire a new pair of eyes with which to see the reality of care (or uncare) as experienced by people with dementia" (Barnett 1993).

It is important never to lose sight of the emotional disturbances caused by a dementing condition. For genuine and effective care to take place we need to imagine what the person with dementia may be feeling: loss, grief, anger, confusion, disempowerment, anguish, isolation, loss of identity and an inability to think or understand the world as one used to. Mappers must also be aware of their own needs, as well as those of the persons being cared for, so as to avoid the possibility of projection (attributing one's own attitudes, ideas and beliefs to another).

The DCM method uses two coding frames. The first, Behaviour Category Coding, is a record of what types of activities or inactivities are occurring, in successive five minute time frames. An indication of "well-being" or "ill-being", known as a Care Value, is also noted on a six point scale: +5, +3, +1 (a state of relative well-being), or -1, -3, -5 (a state of relative ill-being).

The second frame keeps a record of any short-lived episodes in which a person with dementia is demeaned or depersonalised in some way; this is known as Personal Detraction Coding. There are five levels of detraction: mild, moderate, severe, very severe, and extreme.

The raw data can be processed in a number of ways. For example, a Behaviour Category Grid shows the distribution of activities and inactivities, and a Care Value Profile shows the distribution of scores on the six point scale opposite (Fig 1).

The practice of DCM enables the observer to attend very closely to many features of the care environment, as well as to record data in coded form. The information collected can then be used to build up a picture of the present care environment. On discussing the findings from the two evaluations, it will become evident that the data collected cannot be separated from other observations made.

Evaluating our observations

In the two day centres we observed, we found much goodwill, warmth, sociability, ease, friendliness, respect and encouragement. Also, the physical environments were pleasant and relaxing. All these aspects were reflected in the concern shown by clients towards care staff, ourselves and each other. Undoubtedly, a high standard of care was being achieved in both places. By the standards of today, then, the centres were well above the norm, and both had a deservedly strong reputation. Their evaluation thus provides some kind of yardstick of how far the new culture in dementia care has advanced.

Our evaluations were carried out by invitation, which indicates the willingness of the centres to put themselves under scrutiny. Probably there were other reasons, too, for requesting a DCM exercise. For example, there may have been a desire for recognition and recommendation; or perhaps it was hoped that the evaluation would help in bringing about changes in relationships between staff and management, or between the centre and the clients.

The findings from both evaluations were remarkably similar, especially in relation to the overall quality of care. For both centres, on both days, the Care Value

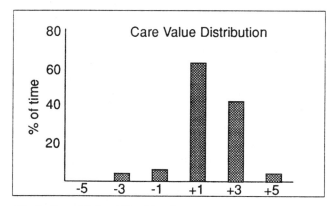

Fig 1: Care Value Distribution

Profiles showed a marked peak at +1; there were relatively few negative Care Values, but also not many +3 or +5. One example is shown in Fig 1 below:

There is certainly cause for encouragement here, and evidence that a new culture of care is beginning to grow. However, in both centres there was evidence to suggest that a plateau may have been reached, and that

investments were being made to keep the status quo. (Evidence to suggest this will be discussed under the headings that follow.) Nevertheless, the potential and opportunities were there, in each place, to develop a more genuinely therapeutic environment.

Care plans and record keeping

Before the evaluations, both centres provided profiles of each person attending. Although these contained valuable information about the clients' background and medical history, they tended to be static. There was no evidence of on-going individual profiles, which could provide more detailed information on a particular person's changing preferences, likes, dislikes, tastes, interests, skills or hobbies, or to give some indication of what might be drawn upon to enhance well-being.

If this type of information were made available to care staff, within the correct bounds of confidentiality, it could facilitate much greater understanding of the clients. Needs could be catered for more appropriately by introducing specific activities based on the interests of those attending the centres, the information being kept on individual profiles which are continually updated.

Minimizing social divisions

During the evaluations there often seemed to be an unintentional "us" and "them" division occurring between care staff and clients, both in attitudes and patterns of action.

It is doubtful, for example, whether staff need to wear uniforms. Comfortable and appropriate dress would seem quite sufficient and more homely. Care staff did not share mealtimes, or social and relaxing moments, on an equal basis with the persons they cared for. During DCM evaluations mappers attempt, as much as possible, to blend into the care environment. This enables the people present to relax more, giving mappers the chance to gain a greater understanding and a much richer insight into each person's life experiences and preferences. More than that, it is often the case that areas of concern regarding health, personal difficulties, insecurities, or particular dependency needs are revealed.

The key point, then, is this. While many practical care tasks have, of course, to be carried out, they can be done in a way that either enhances or diminishes personhood. Being with each other "person to person" (Kitwood and Bredin 1991) can reduce the difference between staff and those being cared for. There is a need to develop the ability simply to "be" with persons who have dementia, on an equal human level.

Giving the opportunity for choice

Making choices and initiating action are key elements of personhood. Conversely, lack of choice can slowly drain away parts of a person's independence that could have remained strong. This process can occur so gradually and with such very small incidents, that it can easily go unnoticed. Our findings suggest that failure to give choice is sometimes tied up with matters of convenience. The small incidents in which choice was denied related to things like music, TV, activities, food or seating. During the mapping we could directly observe the denial of choice causing dejection and a lack of purpose.

A person with dementia may of course be dependent in many different ways. It is, however, the skills and abilities that remain which need to be kept alive, and care givers are in a position to enable this to happen. Helping a person to make choices can give them a sense of being valued, of being heard and of being significant in the world.

Balance of activities

In both centres the practicalities of care were generally dealt with efficiently and with goodwill, but this was out of balance with other much needed provision. For example, gentle exercise, sensory stimulation, handicrafts, games, self-care, expressive or creative pursuits, featured to only a small extent. Also, the clients were given very little opportunity to engage in work or work-like activities.

In neither centre did there appear to be a range of activities genuinely suited to the clients. One centre seemed to have a bias towards the intellect, as if cognition was of extreme importance. In the other centre, there was a tendency towards order, with fixed and planned group activities. In neither place was there much space for individual choice.

While concentration on intellectual stimulation can sometimes be encouraging or entertaining, in some instances we found it served only as a reminder of abilities clients have lost. One woman even made this point in her own personal protest, declaring "Why do you keep reminding us of things we can no longer do?" For overall well-being the emphasis needs, then, to be taken away from the intellect: "Care-giving in dementia emphasises that, in the absence of cures or treatments for dementia, happiness and the individual's capacity for it are more acceptable goals than improved cognition" (Jones & Mieson 1992).

Planned activities may be convenient, but we found the outcome, in some cases, was frustration, boredom, and irritation for the clients. In other words, a culture of "convenient care" had been established, especially in the second of the two centres. Thus individual needs, abilities, talents and tastes were not catered for as well as they might have been. Such a controlled environment could hinder the possibility of personal development and create greater dependency. Also, paradoxically, it can cause unnecessary pressures on care staff.

Feeding the senses

The evaluations revealed that sense-related needs were not being met nearly enough to enhance well-being. In both centres there was evident skill, as shown for example in a beautiful episode of hand massage. Overall, however, there were only isolated incidents of sense-related interaction. Much of the time, the use of the senses to enhance well-being was avoided. Thus, neither centre had found ways to respond appropriately to this area of need. It may be that if staff were more able to meet these needs in themselves, they would more readily understand how important this is for others.

The "multi-sensory" approach, whereby a room is equipped with apparatus to facilitate relaxation and lower levels of agitation (Long & Haig 1992) has achieved some very positive results. However, it is not necessary to have a specially equipped room or indeed elaborate or expensive apparatus. Manufacturers of multi-sensory equipment are now beginning to recognise this, in their move to accommodate home care needs. Everyday materials such as fabrics (natural and man-made), making use of gentle sounds, fragrances, or massage therapy to stimulate all the senses, together with our own simple human resources, can be used creatively so that the effects can be shared and be of benefit to all, at any time, and in any place. Neither centre seemed to have absorbed this simple message.

Promoting independence

In the course of our observations we often found that care staff were doing too much for the clients. Again, the danger is that this could slowly drain away independence. In many care situations there is a natural and unintentional tendency to overprotect. For the new culture to develop, though, there is a need to be more aware of situations where this may occur, so that "convenient" practices are not adopted so readily.

Much goodwill was shown by clients towards care staff and ourselves. Clients often offered to help with practical tasks, for example, but these offers were not always recognised or taken up. Such an offer can be meant as a gift, a way of saying "thank you"; it is also a sign of someone striving to maintain usefulness, dignity and independence in a world where these things can so easily be lost.

"The prime task is that of doing positive 'person-work', so as to enable the person with dementia to be and remain a full participant in our shared humanity" (Kitwood 1993a).

Support through distress

One of the most significant issues arising from the evaluations was that those in real need or in some distress sometimes received less care, rather than more. When incidents of distress were attended to, interactions were often very short-lived, lasting typically less than one minute; in some cases this left the person even more disturbed. Attempts were often made to ignore or "jolly along" persons in distress. Reacting like this can deny someone the chance to express powerful emotions, and may create feelings of invalidation and disempowerment.

The main reason for not meeting a person's emotional needs may be a lack of confidence and resourcefulness at the human level; an inability to deal with personal and intimate feelings. If this is the case, then ways must be found to overcome these difficulties. It may be that staff should recognise their own and each other's needy selves, so that they do not negatively impress their needs onto those they care for. This is a topic to which I shall return.

Both centres, then, needed to develop skills that would enable care staff to deal with distress. The ability to listen, support and guide a person during distress, and to recognise their feelings as real, is absolutely essential. Naomi Feil, the founder of Validation Therapy, stresses the importance of allowing a person to feel what they are feeling, without distorting, denying or minimizing it (Feil 1982). Or, as Tom Kitwood has put it:

"The crucial issue is not that of adjusting the person with dementia to our everyday reality, but of adjusting ourselves, or 'tuning-in' to his or her emotional reality"(Kitwood 1992).

If distress were really attended to, this would allow more genuine social interaction so that secure, equal and trusting relationships could develop. It could also be one of the most vital means by which dignity and self-esteem can be restored.

Involvement of family carers

Both day centres were somewhat lacking in relation to accommodating family/home carers. Our findings suggest that another kind of "us" and "them" situation existed – that between professionals and family carers. The boundaries between management, care staff and family carers needed to be clarified, so as to create an open and accepting atmosphere, in which unnecessary barriers are eliminated. Any difficulties or concerns that may arise for anyone, could then be identified and addressed appropriately and swiftly to alleviate any misunderstanding.

The involvement of family carers is of great importance at many different levels. The experience and knowledge family carers possess about the person they care for needs to be embraced and included in some way in on-going individual profiles. Also, if ways could be found to enable home carers to be involved voluntarily in some of the activities or events, or in integrating the person they care for into the environment, this could enhance relationships and serve to break down some of the barriers. Jane Kesterton and Paul Cunningham, in chapter 11 on day

care, show how the life of a day centre is enriched when unnecessary barriers are removed. This kind of involvement could help create the all embracing shared care needed, to benefit persons with dementia and all their carers.

Episodes of Malignant Social Psychology

The Personal Detractions (PDs) coded from both evaluations, although still plentiful, were all at the "mild" or "moderate" level. This is a good sign, because it means that significant changes had already occurred. There was, then, some awareness of the depersonalising effects of such episodes – although ideally there would not be any at all.

The centres were remarkably similar, not only in the number of PDs recorded, but also in the particular types. By far the most frequent episodes in both evaluations were those of unresponsiveness (care staff ignoring verbal or expressive communication); speaking about persons with dementia in their presence; and the giving of mildly disparaging remarks or put-downs.

Our findings support the view that the new culture was not yet in place in either centre. There was a need for staff to develop greater awareness about their own inner conflicts and attitudes, so that helpful interventions could be made, even when they were working under pressure. However, information gathered from our evaluations does suggest that attitudes are changing for the better. None of the "severe", "very severe" and "extremely severe" detractions mentioned in the DCM Manual were in evidence, although these were very much part of the old culture of care.

Staff support

Dementia care work, much of the time, can be both physically exhausting and emotionally demanding. All staff in any care environment need a great deal of on-going and consistent support if their efforts are to be genuinely effective. Our evaluations found relatively little support, appreciation, understanding or encouragement between care staff, support workers and managers. In one centre, there were even situations in which care staff were humiliated in public, and instances of staff conflict and disagreement occurred in the view of clients.

While many signs of commitment, dedication and insight were shown on the part of staff, their reactions to certain situations seemed limited by lack of support. There was a need for space to be provided, and time set aside during working hours, so that trust and mutual encouragement could be established. There was also a need for a much fuller briefing and debriefing, so that successes, difficulties and conflicts (both professional and personal), could be openly addressed and discussed in a safe and accepting way.

The experience of evaluating

In our observation of care settings, we have come to appreciate just how important it is for those carrying out evaluations to prepare the care team properly, and give them adequate feedback. Although preparation initially tends to come from management, mappers need to give careful and considerate briefing to the direct care team prior to, throughout and after the evaluation. We ourselves may not, in the past, have done this work as well as we might.

However, we came across some difficulties that generally belonged to the centres themselves, which made evaluating quite stressful for all concerned. Attempts to reassure staff do not always reduce apprehension to a desirable level; even knowing in detail what DCM involves may not be effective in eliminating anxiety. We began to sense that such difficulties arose in part because management and staff still retained some of the attitudes of the old culture, in particular the retention of defences, rather than a spirit of openness. Also, staff morale may have been lowered because the current uncertainties gave them a greater need for support. Under such circumstances existing patterns of defence were probably increased.

The two centres showed rather different responses to the evaluations. One centre readily took on board the recommendations made in the report, and instantly set in place a programme to implement the changes they considered necessary to improve care. A further evaluation was envisaged for a future date, so as to make "before" and "after" comparisons. When we came away from this centre, after the final feedback, we had a strong sense of their gratitude and appreciation.

The other centre's response was not so positive. Here, there was a greater degree of unintended "us" and "them" between clients and the care team, and between direct care staff and management. Also, there was little evidence of constructive staff support, and there seemed to be higher stress levels, even though the staffing ratio was very favourable. Under these conditions, it would be much more difficult to adopt a new culture of care, and much safer and easier to remain on the plateau already attained. Defences against change can be due to present stress, because the changes involved could rock or fragment an already fragile setting. Also, new demands would be placed on people who are near to the limit of their skills. We came away from this centre ourselves carrying some feeling of having been discounted. This may, however, have resulted from some inefficacy on our part.

In both centres, we came across some exceptional examples of good quality care. On many occasions we witnessed strong commitment, dedication, sensitivity and much kindness. However, neither management nor care staff acknowledged to each other the good aspects of what they were doing. In other words, where the new culture was genuinely growing it was not being adequately nurtured.

Grounds for encouragement

The message of the new culture in dementia care is at one level quite simple; care for others as you yourself would wish to be cared for. At another level, though, it is exceedingly complex, because we have to find within ourselves skills and sensitivities far beyond those which are used in the ordinary course of everyday life.

"If we dare to draw closer, dementia care can become a profound and creative experience...as we discover the person who has dementia, we also discover something of ourselves" (Kitwood 1993b).

The DCM method is a powerful tool, which can reveal the extent of the new culture in dementia care. If these two evaluations are any guide, they would suggest that the new culture has begun to take root, but its growth is uneven and spasmodic. It is only when the Care Value Profiles show their peak around the +3 level rather than +1, and when the Behaviour Category Grid shows a really balanced range of activities, that we will be sure that the necessary growth is taking place.

References

Barnett, E. (1993) Observing Care in Detail – The DCM Method, *Alzheimer's Disease Society July Newsletter.*

Feil N (1982) *Validation: The Feil Method.* Edward Feil Productions. Cleveland, Ohio.

Jones GMM, Miesen BML Eds. (1992) *Care Giving in Dementia. Research and Applications.* Tavistock, London.

Kitwood T, Bredin K (1991) *Person to Person: A Guide to the Care of Those with Failing Mental Powers.* Gale Centre Publications, Loughton, Essex.

Kitwood T (1992) Towards a Theory of Dementia Care: Personhood and Well-being. *Ageing and Society* **12** 269-287.

Kitwood T (1993a) *Ageing and Later Life.* Open University Press Course Reader, pp100-106.

Kitwood T (1993b) Discover the Person not the Disease. *Journal of Dementia Care* **1(1)** 16-17.

Long AP, Haig L (1992) How clients benefit from Snoezelen. An explanatory study. *British Journal of Occupational Therapy,* 28, 529-536.

CHAPTER SIXTEEN | Strategies for training and organisational change

BRENDA BOWE
BUZ LOVEDAY

Various strategies for bringing about the wide range of changes the new culture of dementia care demands are discussed. Both informal and formal training methods are examined, focusing on ways of meeting the needs of individual caregivers. The organisational context is discussed, and the necessary commitment to the new culture from both local and senior managers is considered.

Many people who are committed to the new culture of dementia care are looking for ways of putting its principles into practice. The more we realise the potential inherent in new models of care (Kitwood & Bredin 1992a), the more destructive the old approaches seem to be. We become acutely aware of the poor care we may have practised, managed or witnessed. We realise the damage this has caused: the erosion of personhood which we had perhaps thought we had no power to prevent. We now feel a sense of urgency to start to put things right.

We each have various strategies at our disposal which we can use to help influence the type of care which is given to people with dementia. The carer who joins with others and speaks out against the poor care practices his relative has received; the manager who treats her own staff as real persons and helps them understand the needs of those they are caring for; the careworker who, through her own approach, demonstrates to her colleagues what a difference person-centred care can make: each has some power to bring about positive changes. Each has their own important contribution to make. And every change, however small, moves us further towards establishing the new culture of dementia care.

Spectrum of changes

There is a wide spectrum of necessary changes, ranging from the details of care received by each individual to major organisational restructuring. Changes at every point of the spectrum are important, and it is essential to recognise the impact that even a small change can have on the quality of life of an individual with dementia. For Ethel, it could make all the difference in the world that she is now given the time and assistance

to eat her own lunch, rather than being spoon-fed by a hurried staff member. For Harry, a new feeling of self-worth could develop because staff, having discovered that he used to be a keen gardener, ask for his help and advice in planting out seedlings in the day centre garden. These changes, affecting people's day to day lives, are both urgent and relatively easy to achieve. They do not have major budgeting implications, nor do they take a long time to introduce.

There is no organisational restructuring which could bring about a new culture of care if the caregivers involved are still entrenched in the same old attitudes and approach. However wonderful the new, purpose-built nursing home, if people with dementia are still seen as difficult and demanding; if Louise is still called a "naughty girl" when she doesn't want to have a bath, or Michael gets told to sit down every time he stands up, life for individual people with dementia will not have changed enough.

Changes at an individual level, then, must happen prior to or alongside any organisational changes which are made. But changes on a broader scale are essential too. If the new practices relating to care given to individuals are not reflected in the policies and procedures of an organisation, the occurrence of such changes at an individual level is left to chance, and ultimately may not be consistent or sustained.

Strategies for change

Individuals across the country who are working towards the new culture have found numerous strategies which can help to improve care practices and attitudes. The new culture, tapping as it does into our intrinsic human qualities, makes immediate sense, even while it challenges us quite profoundly. But, of course, the old culture has a lot going for it too, in the security of the familiar, the simplicity of generalisations, the distancing of others to protect our vulnerable selves. It is not easy for people to leave all this behind. We must realise that we cannot bring about the new culture overnight; it cannot simply be donned like a new coat. We must be prepared to work slowly and persistently, chipping away at the old culture as we lay, and then build on, the foundations of the new one.

So how are we to bring about the necessary changes? Training is often seen as a key strategy, and some approaches and methods for training in the new culture are considered later in this chapter.

In addition to formal training, which might take the shape of workshops or courses, there are many kinds of informal training which can be carried out by anyone in the care setting. This could involve staff and managers "role-modelling" the person-centred approach; managers giving constructive supervision, advice and support; a whole staff group sharing ideas at staff meetings; careworkers offering feedback to each other; staff and managers listening to and learning from carers. Learning can happen in many ways, and the most important teachers are people with dementia themselves. If we can be open to learning from them, each individual who has dementia will educate and inform us about their needs.

Such informal training is crucial in the process of bringing about change and must be practised in addition to any formal training which is offered. Good communication is also essential. The same clear message needs to be given to caregivers and managers at all levels of an organisation, and this message needs to be constantly repeated, using existing forums and, as necessary, developing new ones. Another integral component is for each staff member and manager to take responsibility and ownership of how they influence the quality of life of those in their care. Old models of care did not acknowledge this influence, and so if staff are to recognise the importance of changing their practices, they must first become aware of their own power.

For any organisation which is using such strategies to try to bring about changes, there will be a need to examine progress and the effects of these new approaches. Dementia Care Mapping (Kitwood & Bredin 1992b) is a method of evaluating care from the perspective of the person with dementia, and thus provides us with crucial feedback about how our care affects the person receiving it. The findings can enable staff to develop and modify care in line with individual needs, and thus Dementia Care Mapping can, in itself, be an important tool for facilitating change.

Training

The majority of training opportunities for caregivers tend to be provided through externally run training courses. Such courses undoubtedly have value, but there are obvious difficulties for those who go on such courses in coming back to the workplace and attempting to make changes. We each have the power to change our own attitude and approach; indeed, this is the most essential first step. But it can be much harder to try to change others. For many who, through training, feel able to change their own approach, there can be a sense of frustration and powerlessness when confronted with the unchanged care practices of their

colleagues. If externally run training courses are to play a part in promoting organisational changes, we must find a way of supporting and empowering these individuals once they return to the workplace. Alternatively, if we bring the training into the care setting, we can involve everyone who works there, ensuring that the same information and opportunities are given to all so that everyone can move forward together.

Training needs

Bringing training into the care setting also offers the opportunity to get in touch with individual needs. Each organisation which cares for people with dementia might have different problems and concerns. And within the care setting, each member of the staff team may have different skills, attitudes and experiences. Training must respect the uniqueness of each care setting and of the individuals who work in it. In this way, training itself can be person-centred - a necessary pre-requisite when the aim of this training is to promote person-centred care practice.

Those who work with people with dementia often have much to say when asked what help they need in relation to their work. Some of this might relate to their difficulties or concerns about individual clients. Some might relate more to issues of staff group dynamics or personal problems. There might also be a need for assistance or information which can help them connect with the experiences of those they are caring for. It is very important that staff are given the opportunity to express these needs and that training, when given, represents them.

Many people, for a variety of reasons, might be resistant to the idea of training. Those who have been working with people with dementia for a long time (within the old culture) might feel they know everything there is to know, and are comfortable with the previously accepted ways of doing things. Others might be affected by the low status which their work was often accorded within the old culture, and not feel motivated to put any more effort into their jobs.

We are demanding a lot of any training to ask it to break through this sort of resistance. It is essential that the training itself makes an effort to meet the staff where they are, recognising their existing skills and experience as well as their problems, and being highly relevant to their day to day situation.

In discussing their training needs, there tend to be many issues and concerns which different staff groups working with people with dementia share. The need for factual information about dementia is often seen as a priority, together with help on practical skills such as communication and groupwork. It is evident that staff often have many gaps in their knowledge and understanding and this can cause them frustrations and problems in doing their work. The old culture had many unfair expectations of care workers, including the belief that goodwill and common sense alone were the only requirements for the job.

In researching training needs, there is also much to be learnt about the assumptions and beliefs which staff may hold. Trainers may be asked for help on "managing problem behaviour" or "how to make them do what you want them to do". It is evident that the assumptions inherent in such requests - for example, that the behaviour of people with dementia is meaningless and needs to be controlled - must also be addressed in training. These assumptions give rise to the attitudes which inform care practice, and these attitudes are the crucial focus for change. The learning of information and new skills will go some way towards raising awareness and helping workers change their attitude towards people with dementia. But, in addition, we will need to devote specific time to questioning, challenging and discussing attitudes through the use of experiential training exercises.

Training methods

Since the need for facts about dementia is often presented by staff as a priority, trainers need to address this. However, it is important that such facts are not taught in a way which colludes with a problem-focused, de-humanising view of dementia. Of course, people may need to gain some understanding of neurological impairment and the symptoms which can result, but we should always emphasise how care practices, too, can play a part in increasing or decreasing the effects of these symptoms. We also need to help careworkers understand individual differences, rather than seeing people with dementia as all the same. We need to focus on strengths, as well as symptoms, helping staff appreciate that people with dementia can be assisted to live fully in spite of their disability.

The methods used to present such facts will vary according to the abilities and particular needs of the group being trained. It is always important to help people learn from each other, and validate the existing knowledge which people may have, while gently challenging incorrect facts and assumptions which hail from the old culture. Trainers can use methods such as brainstorms, quizzes and discussions to encourage participants to share their knowledge in a non-threatening way.

Trainers will also need to present new facts, perhaps using a combination of verbal presentation, handouts and audio-visual material. For participants who are not used to formal learning situations, it is important that the presentation of facts does not take the form of a long, dry lecture, but is lively and engaging.

Training to assist in the development of new skills is another important area. In order to learn new skills, people need to be given an opportunity to practice them. Role play can be an extremely useful technique which, in addition to giving people an opportunity to try out and receive feedback on new skills, gives them a chance to "be" the person with dementia and view these approaches and techniques from the receiving end. Case studies, or similar group exercises where people can work together to gain an understanding of a situation and perhaps find an appropriate response, are also an opportunity for trainees to broaden their understanding. In such exercises, participants can begin to apply what they have learnt, thus moving one step closer to practising the new skills in real life. Ongoing training can also give careworkers the opportunity to feed back on how their new knowledge and skills are entering into their day-to-day practice, and to discuss any difficulties which have arisen.

Probably the most important focus for training is on attitudes and assumptions. We learn most powerfully through our own experiences (Hobbs 1992), and training exercises can create opportunities for such experiential learning, getting people thinking, talking and feeling. Exercises can be used, for example, to help caregivers realise what the experience of dementia might be like. Such an exercise might involve asking people to consider how they would feel and respond in the kind of situations which people with dementia face every day. How would they feel, for example, if they were lost in an unfamiliar place where they didn't speak the language or know the customs? Or if they were confronted by an apparent stranger who told them they needed a bath? This can be an important step in people recognising, perhaps for the first time, what might be happening in the world of the person with dementia.

Training exercises can also be used to break down the "us and them" barrier (Kitwood & Bredin 1992c) which can often get in the way of person-to-person contact between careworkers and people with dementia. One way of starting to overcome this barrier is to help people step into the shoes of "them". For example, participants can be asked to discuss this question: "What do you think you might be like if you got dementia?" People can often realise that what they had previously viewed as "problem behaviour" might well be the way they, too, would respond to the constraints of their environment or the frustrations of their condition.

In another training exercise, participants can be assisted to confront and ultimately to discard old ways of thinking, by sharing all the labels and generalisations they might have heard or used about people with dementia. This can be a powerful reminder of our own prejudices. Participants can feel shocked as they realise how they have condemned people and consider the effects that such generalisations can have, by keeping people with dementia at a distance and labelling them as somehow inferior to ourselves. Care staff who take part in this exercise can realise that their own negative expectations can turn into a self-fulfilling prophecy as the people with dementia they care for react to what is assumed and expected of them.

If we encourage people to learn from their own feelings and experiences, we are also helping them to get in touch with their own personhood (Rogers 1967). Too often, those involved in caring work have, through lack of support and recognition, had to protect themselves by creating a barrier between themselves and those they are caring for. Their true feelings and natural responses might be buried deeply, at least until they leave the workplace at the end of the day. If careworkers are to begin to drop their defences, it is crucial that we find a way of providing them with the necessary support.

Many different tools can be used in training to promote discussion and learning, from videos to role plays, case studies to games, thinking about both real life situations and imaginary scenarios. If training is interactive and varied it is much more likely to hold people's attention and engage them in the process of change (Jelfs 1982).

Training exercises can be devised in order to meet exactly the needs of the group receiving the training. Training which is tailor-made in this way can be particularly effective in connecting with individual attitudes and experiences. But creating new materials can be very time consuming, and for this reason, those involved in delivering training often need to select and adapt from the wide range of existing material to suit the needs of the individual caregivers or organisation.

It needs to be noted, however, that much available material tends to approach dementia from a problem-centred or medical perspective; for example, it is much more common for videos to show interviews with carers talking about their difficulties, than to show what life is like for the person with dementia and what might help to make things better for them. Each side of the story needs to be told, but what is important is to find a balance between the two. We cannot learn how best to care for people with dementia if we never see the situation from their perspective. For this reason it is important to devise or search out training materials which illustrate and reinforce a person-centred approach. Training and its desired goal can be totally undermined if different, contradictory approaches are promoted with the same staff group.

Change in the organisation

Local management
In developing a training strategy, it is important to consider not just the content to be included and the methods to be used, but also the larger context within which the training is to take place. We have already stated that changes need to be reinforced at an organisational level. It is the first level of the organisational hierarchy –the on-site management group – which has the most immediate influence on care practices. As part of any programme of change, it is crucial to consider the needs of these managers: What will the implications of such changes be for them? What is their commitment to the new culture? What is their own current understanding and awareness? What are their priorities?

It is important that managers are given the same opportunities as staff for training which helps them develop their insight and understanding about the needs of people with dementia. If they are to positively influence care practice, it is crucial that managers role-model the approach which is being advocated. The way they communicate with people with dementia in their care sets an example for staff. The attitudes and opinions they express are often very influential.

Managers can also benefit from training which looks specifically at needs and issues related to their role. In particular, such training can focus on strategies which they can use to implement and reinforce a person-centred approach to the care of people with dementia. From a management perspective, there are certain changes which need to be made if a person-centred approach is to be adopted. The emphasis within care settings needs to move away from task-orientated routines and towards a more flexible system which puts the clients' needs above those of the organisation.

Perhaps a first step is to look at both the quantity and quality of face-to-face time that staff actually spend with those they are caring for. There is also a need to minimise any contradictory expectations imposed on staff: if the value of communicating and building relationships is being promoted, it is both inconsistent and damaging for a manager to interrupt a conversation between a worker and a client to tell the worker to go and fold the laundry, for example.

Managers need to make clear exactly what is being expected of staff. For example, is the worker's role primarily to address the client's practical needs, or is the worker also expected to offer emotional support? It would seem that the latter is essential if the intention is to provide person-centred care, but this means that managers must also be prepared to offer staff a deeper level of support than may have been necessary within the old culture. If staff are giving more of themselves to those they are caring for, through their empathy, energy and creativity, they in turn will have emotional needs which must be addressed or they will switch off or burn out. In addition to the support which managers can offer, it might also be necessary for staff to have access to support groups or individual counselling. In essence, managers and organisations need to adopt a person-centred approach to their staff.

Organisational commitment

Organisationally, the implications of the new culture of dementia care need to be carefully considered. Firstly, the organisation must publicly own the new approach, but it is not enough simply to make mission statements and use the right jargon. It is not enough just to run a training course or have Dementia Care Mapping carried out if this is merely a token gesture and is not followed through. The organisation needs to ensure that this new approach is practised. The new expectations need to be made explicit to employees at all levels.

This means that recruitment procedures, personnel specifications and job descriptions must all incorporate the person-centred approach as a key component. Supervision and appraisal must be used to monitor care practices and consistently make clear what is acceptable and what isn't. And, of course, the organisation must provide its employees with whatever resources are necessary for the new approach to become a reality.

Those who are attempting to encourage organisations to adopt the new approaches might well encounter resistance. Perhaps the biggest selling point of the new culture is that its implications are not primarily financial. Indeed, there is a great deal which can be achieved without any extra expenditure.

Yet organisations can be extremely defensive about preserving the status quo. Senior managers who have little, if any, contact with service users are often out of touch with the details of care practices and the well-being of individual clients, particularly if no complaints have been made through official channels. Furthermore, in this era of many changes within Social Services and the National Health Service, it is understandable that there can be a reluctance to embark on yet another programme of change, particularly one which is not required by legislation. But even while we understand some of this organisational resistance, we must work to combat it, advocating on behalf of those individuals who tend to be given no voice.

The new culture of dementia care is growing in strength, but even though we use our most creative strategies, its progress can often be slow. Anyone working to bring about these changes is going to feel frustrated at times. Frustrated at the entrenched attitudes which seem impossible to shift; with the resistance we encounter at every level; with the low priority which is often accorded to the care of people with dementia.

But if we focus on the situation from a different perspective we can become more optimistic as we realise just how achievable the new culture really is. Primarily, the need is for changed attitudes and practice, which does not necessarily indicate increased budgets and new buildings; thus financial considerations need not be an obstacle nor an excuse for inaction. Furthermore, the old culture is not innately ours - its principles have been learnt by those who practise it and in the same way they can be un-learnt, as an alternative is offered in their place.

And finally we must consider the rewards inherent in the new culture, not just for people with dementia, but for those who care for them: the increased job satisfaction as staff become enablers rather than controllers, relate to persons rather than to problems and feel both appreciated and empowered in their work. And whatever strategies we use to assist the new culture on its way in, ultimately it will be our own belief in its value which gives us the commitment to succeed.

References

Hobbs T (Ed) (1992) *Experiential Training - Practical Guidelines*. Tavistock/Routledge, London.

Jelfs M (1982) *Manual for Action - Techniques to enable groups engaged in action for change to increase their effectiveness*. Action Resources Group c/o 13 Mornington Grove, London E3.

Kitwood T and Bredin K (1992a) *Person to Person – A guide to the care of those with failing mental powers*. Gale Centre Publications, Loughton, Essex.

Kitwood T and Bredin K (1992b) A new approach to the evaluation of dementia care. *Journal of Advances in Health and Nursing Care* **1(5)** 41-60.

Kitwood T and Bredin K (1992c) Towards a Theory of Dementia Care: Personhood and Well-being. *Ageing and Society* **12** 269-287.

Rogers C (1967) *On Becoming a Person - A Therapist's View of Psychotherapy*. Constable, London.

Index

Abuse 20
Activity 19, 57, 66-69, 72
Aggression 56, 59
Alienation 9, 11
Asylums 7-9
Baking 57
Behaviour
  "problem"/challenging 10, 21, 36-38
Behaviour modification 21
Bestialisation 7
Burn-out 10, 22
Care package 7, 17
Care plans 71
Carers 10, 13, 15-18, 20, 21, 36-37, 49-53, 54, 55, 57, 59-61,62-65, 73
Communication 10, 12-14, 15-18, 24-29, 32-33, 66
Competence 10, 24-29
Continence 13, 22, 56
Culture 7-11
Day care 17, 54-57
Dementia care mapping 24, 55, 70-74
Disability 8, 10, 13, 16,
Domus units 20
Environment 8, 13-14, 19, 56-57, 59-60, 70-74
Family carers 15-18, 20-21, 36-37, 49-53, 54-55, 57, 59-61, 62-65, 73
Genetics 44-48
Gentle teaching 21
Home care 17
Hospital 17
Incontinence 13, 22, 56
Infantilisation 18, 28
Institutions 7-11, 20, 69
Language 24-29
Learning 14
Learning difficulties/disabilities 20-21
Long-term care 18
Management 22, 78-79
Manicure 57
Meals 9, 55, 56, 57
Medicalisation 7
Medical science 8
Memory 12-14
Mindfulness 33-34

Mini-Mental State Examination 25
Moralisation 7
Music 51
Neglect 20
Neighbourhood centre 17
Normalisation 21
Norton Scale 25
Occupation 66-69
Ordinary living 21
Organisations 10, 22, 36, 38, 75-79
Paranoia 13
Personality 8, 13-14, 16, 27-29, 30-34
Physical care 9, 33, 36, 37
Prime carer 54-55
Psychoanalysis 8
Psychotherapy 21
Quality assurance 22
Quality control 22
Reality orientation 19-20
Record keeping 71
Reminiscence 20
Research 9, 15-16, 22-23, 24, 44-48
Resolution therapy 20
Rights 14, 30
  and risk 18
Risk 18, 57
Senses 66-69, 72
Sexual abuse 38
Sexuality 35-39
Shared care 15-18
Sheltered housing 58-61
Social psychology 9, 73
Social role valorisation 21
Spirituality 40-43
Staff needs 10, 22, 36, 38, 73, 76
Stage theories 10, 12-14
Stimulation 19
Toileting 9, 56
Training 8, 57, 61, 65, 67-68, 75-79
Uniforms 57
Validation therapy 20
Vegetative state 12, 66
Violence 56
Volunteers 62-65